# Oxford Handbook of
# Emergencies in Clinical Radiology

Edited by

## Richard Graham MA FRCR

Specialist Registrar in Radiology, John Radcliffe and
Churchill Hospitals, Oxford, UK
Lecturer in Medicine, Hertford College, University of
Oxford, Oxford, UK

and

## Ferdia Gallagher MA MRCP FRCR

Cancer Research UK and Royal College of Radiologists
Clinical Research Training Fellow, University of Cambridge
and CRUK Cambridge Research Institute, Cambridge, UK
Honorary Specialist Registrar, Addenbrooke's Hospital,
Cambridge, UK

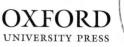

OXFORD
UNIVERSITY PRESS

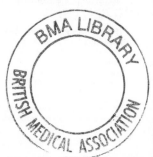

# OXFORD
UNIVERSITY PRESS

Great Clarendon Street, Oxford OX2 6DP

Oxford University Press is a department of the University of Oxford.
It furthers the University's objective of excellence in research, scholarship,
and education by publishing worldwide in

Oxford New York

Auckland Cape Town Dar es Salaam Hong Kong Karachi
Kuala Lumpur Madrid Melbourne Mexico City Nairobi
New Delhi Shanghai Taipei Toronto

With offices in

Argentina Austria Brazil Chile Czech Republic France Greece
Guatemala Hungary Italy Japan Poland Portugal Singapore
South Korea Switzerland Thailand Turkey Ukraine Vietnam

Oxford is a registered trade mark of Oxford University Press
in the UK and in certain other countries

Published in the United States
by Oxford University Press Inc., New York

© Oxford University Press 2009

The moral rights of the author have been asserted
Database right Oxford University Press (maker)

First published 2009

British Library Cataloguing in Publication Data
Data available

Library of Congress Cataloging in Publication Data
Data available.

Typeset by Cepha Imaging Private Ltd., Bangalore, India
Printed in China
on acid-free paper through
Asia Pacific Offset Limited

ISBN 978-0-19-923843-9

10 9 8 7 6 5 4 3 2 1

Oxford University Press makes no representation, express or implied, that the drug dosages
in this book are correct. Readers must therefore always check the product information
and clinical procedures with the most up-to-date published product information and data
sheets provided by the manufacturers and the most recent codes of conduct and safety
regulations. The authors and the publishers do not accept responsibility or legal liability for
any errors in the text or for the misuse or misapplication of material in this work.

▶ Except where otherwise stated, drug doses and recommendations are for the non-
pregnant adult who is not breast-feeding.

# Dedication

To Bessie, Anita and Ciara.

# Foreword

This is a very valuable contribution to the literature and will become a standard reference book for radiologists young and old. Indeed all imaging departments should have several copies close to hand in case of emergencies. The market was crying out for just such a book, especially as Saxton and Strickland's 'Procedures' and Ansell's 'Complication' books have now become obsolete. Of course, with the rapid changes in technology and guidelines, even this book will age quite quickly too. But it was good to see the authors anticipate the future by considering CT as the initial investigation for chest pain (the triple rule out – myocardial infarction, aortic dissection and pulmonary embolism).

This young and energetic cast of editors and authors has assembled an extraordinary amount of useful facts within a short space. By judicious use of lists and a minimum of free text, they make it an ideal cramming book before FRCR and other 'board type' examination. It may also prove popular amongst medical students and allied health professionals (radiographers, technicians, etc).

As an editor with relatively fixed views on style, there are very few terms that jar on the eyes. Just occasionally the reader may get confused by which type of 'scan' is being referred to! And I am never quite sure what a 'modality' is. But these are minor quibbles from an ageing dinosaur. This is a modern book with a modern feel.

All in all, this team has done a marvellous job. I wish the book (and its subsequent revised editions) well.

Adrian K Dixon
Cambridge

# Preface

This book has arisen out of our own experiences as radiology trainees and those of our colleagues. Trainees are often daunted by the breadth of knowledge required to successfully manage an emergency radiology service, particularly when on-call; radiology has equivalent subspecialties for almost every branch of medicine and emergency radiology is an essential component of each. A very high proportion of patients who enter the emergency department will undergo some form of imaging before leaving hospital and these tests will often be central in determining their management. It is unusual for a patient to undergo emergency surgery without prior imaging and cranial CT is now crucial to clinical decision-making following head trauma.

Consequently, there has been a steady increase in demand for emergency imaging, which can put huge pressure on radiology departments. This pressure is also experienced by trainees who are frequently on the front line of emergency radiology on-call and while there are many excellent radiology textbooks there has been no single, easily assessable text that provides guidance on how to successfully manage radiology on-calls. It is from these observations made by ourselves, friends and colleagues that the idea of this handbook was born.

The emergency radiologist faces two questions with each emergency case: what is the correct imaging modality to answer the clinical question and how should this be performed to optimize the imaging information obtained? The answers to these questions are often not straightforward and in the pressure of the emergency setting, when time is crucial, incorrect imaging may result leading to suboptimal patient management. This book is a guide for the emergency radiologist as to which imaging is most appropriate in what circumstance, how best to perform it, and how to interpret the results. In all cases, discussion with an experienced clinician will help to optimize the diagnostic power of the investigation.

*Emergencies in Clinical Radiology* is intended as a readily accessible reference for specialist trainees in clinical radiology as well as radiographers. In addition, it will be of use to other hospital specialists involved in the emergency care of patients as it provides advice on which radiological investigation to request in a particular clinical setting. The text lists imaging strategies for frequently presenting complaints and common conditions, including the relative merits of each modality and advice on how they may be optimized. It also discusses the expected radiological findings to aid interpretation of these tests.

We hope the use of this book will help all those involved in emergency imaging and will ultimately enhance patient care. We would value any feedback to improve future editions.

RG
FG
2008

# Ackowledgements

We would like to thank OUP for their help in the preparation of this book, especially Chris Reid and Fiona Goodgame who have been very supportive throughout the project. We would also like to thank Professor Adrian Dixon for writing the foreword to the book.

Above all, we are indebted to our many teachers, students, and patients, all of whom have taught us everything we know.

# Contents

# Abbreviations

| | |
|---|---|
| ↑ | increases |
| ↓ | decreases |
| +C | plus contrast medium |
| +Gd | plus gadolinium chelate (MRI contrast medium) |
| A&E | accident and emergency department |
| AAST | American Association for the Surgery of Trauma |
| ABLS | adult basic life support |
| ACA | Anterior Cerebral Artery |
| ACS | acute coronary syndrome |
| ADC | apparent diffusion coefficient |
| AED | automated external defibrillator |
| ALI | acute lung injury |
| ALS | advanced life support |
| AP | anteroposterior |
| APC | activated protein C |
| APH | ante-partum haemorrhage |
| ATLS | Advanced Trauma Life Support |
| AV | arteriovenous |
| AVM | arteriovenous malformation |
| AXR | abdominal radiograph |
| BA | basilar artery |
| BLS | basic life support |
| BM | blood glucose (Boehringer Mannheim test) |
| BMT | bone marrow transplant |
| BPM | beats per minute |
| BTS | British Thoracic Society |
| CBD | common bile duct |
| CCA | common carotid artery |
| CECT | contrast-enhanced CT |
| CK-MB | MB isoenzyme of creatine kinase |
| CMV | cytomegalovirus |
| CNS | central nervous system |
| CPR | cardiopulmonary resuscitation |
| CSF | cerebrospinal fluid |
| C-spine | cervical spine |
| CT | computed tomography |

| | |
|---|---|
| CTA | computed tomographic angiography |
| CTPA | CT pulmonary angiography |
| CTV | CT venography |
| CVC | central venous catheter |
| CXR | chest radiograph |
| DM | diabetes mellitus |
| DOB | Date of Birth |
| DUS | Doppler ultrasound |
| DWI | diffusion weighted imaging (on MRI) |
| EAMs | external auditory meati |
| ECG | electrocardiogram |
| EDH | extradural haematoma |
| ERCP | endoscopic retrograde cholangiopancreatography |
| ETT | endotracheal tube |
| EVAR | endovascular aneurysm repair |
| FAST | focused assessment with sonography in trauma |
| FB | foreign body |
| FBC | full blood count |
| FLAIR | fluid-attenuated inversion recovery |
| Fr | French catheter scale (outer diameter in mm x 3) |
| FS | fat-suppressed imaging (on MRI) |
| G | gauge of needle |
| GA | general anaesthetic |
| GCS | Glasgow Coma Score |
| GFR | glomerular filtration rate |
| GI | gastrointestinal |
| GU | genitourinary |
| Hb | Haemoglobin |
| HDU | high-dependency unit |
| HF | heart failure |
| HIV | human immunodeficiency virus |
| HRCT | high-resolution computed tomography |
| HRT | Hormone Replacement Therapy |
| HSV | herpes simplex virus |
| HU | Hounsfield units |
| ICA | internal carotid artery |
| ICP | intracranial pressure |
| IJV | internal jugular vein |
| IM | intramuscular |
| INR | international normalized ratio |

| IRMER | Ionizing radiation (medical exposures regulation) |
| ITU | intensive therapy unit |
| IV | intravenous |
| IVC | inferior vena cava |
| IVU | intravenous urography |
| LBO | large bowel obstruction |
| LFTs | liver function tests |
| LMWH | low molecular weight heparin |
| LP | lumbar puncture |
| LV | left ventricle |
| MAC | mycobacterium avium complex |
| MCA | middle cerebral artery |
| MCUG | micturating cystourethrogram |
| MDCT | multidetector CT (e.g. 64-slice CT) |
| MDT | multidisciplinary team (meeting) |
| MI | myocardial infarction |
| MIP | maximum intensity projection images |
| MPR(s) | multiplanar reformatted image(s) |
| MR(I) | magnetic resonance (imaging) |
| MRA | magnetic resonance angiography |
| MRCP | magnetic resonance cholangiopancreatography |
| MRSA | methicillin-resistant *Staphylococcus Aureus* |
| MRV | magnetic resonance venogram |
| NAI | non-accidental injury |
| NEC | necrotizing enterocolitis |
| NECT | non-enhanced CT (i.e. without contrast medium) |
| NG(T) | nasogastric (tube) |
| NICE | National Institute for Health and Clinical Excellence |
| NOE | naso-orbitoethmoid |
| NPV | negative predictive value |
| NSAIDs | non-steroidal anti-inflammatory drugs |
| NSTEMI | non-ST elevation myocardial infarction |
| OCP | oral contraceptive pill |
| OM | occipitomental |
| PA | posteroanterior |
| PACS | picture archiving and communication system |
| PC | phase contrast (imaging) |
| PCA | posterior cerebral artery |
| PCI | percutaneous coronary intervention |
| PCP | pneumocystis pneumonia |

| PE | pulmonary embolism |
|---|---|
| PEA | pulseless electrical activity |
| PET | positron emission tomography |
| PICC(s) | peripherally inserted central catheter(s) |
| PIOPEDII | Prospective investigation of pulmonary embolism diagnosis II |
| PO | *per os* (by mouth) |
| PPH | post-partum haemorrhage |
| PPV | positive predictive value |
| PR | *per rectum* |
| PUL | pregnancy of unknown location |
| PV | *per vaginam* (by the vagina) |
| RCR | Royal College of Radiologists |
| RSV | respiratory synsyctial virus |
| RTA | road traffic accident |
| rtPA | recombinant tissue plasminogen activator |
| SAH | subarachnoid haemorrhage |
| SBO | small bowel obstruction |
| SDH | subdural haemorrhage |
| SI | signal intensity |
| SLE | systemic lupus erythematosus |
| SMA | superior mesenteric artery |
| SMV | superior mesenteric vein |
| SOL | space-occupying lesion |
| STEMI | ST elevation myocardial infarction |
| STIR | short tau inversion recovery imaging (on MRI) |
| SUFE | slipped upper femoral epiphysis |
| SVC | superior vena cava |
| SXR | skull radiograph |
| $T_1$ | $T_1$-weighted imaging (on MRI) |
| $T_2$ | $T_2$-weighted imaging (on MRI) |
| TA | transabdominal |
| TAUS | transabdominal US |
| TB | tuberculosis |
| TCC | transitional cell carcinoma |
| TED | thromboembolic deterrent |
| TIA | transient ischaemic attack |
| TOE | transoesophageal echocardiography |
| TOF | time-of-flight imaging (on MRI) |
| TPN | total parenteral nutrition |
| TV | transvaginal |

| TVUS | transvaginal ultrasound |
|------|-------------------------|
| U&E | urea and electrolytes |
| UAC | umbilical arterial catheter |
| US | ultrasound |
| UTI | urinary tract infection |
| UVC | umbilical venous catheter |
| V/Q | ventilation–perfusion scan |
| VF | ventricular fibrillation |
| VRT | volume rendered technique |
| VSD | ventricular septal defect |
| VT | ventricular tachycardia |
| VUJ | vesico-ureteric junction |
| WL | window level of the displayed image |
| WSCM | water-soluble contrast medium |
| WW | window width of the displayed image |
| ZMC | zygomaticomaxillary complex |

# Contributors

**SK Bobby Agrawal FRCS FRCR**
Consultant Cardiothoracic Radiologist
Papworth Hospital NHS Foundation Trust
Papworth Everard, Cambridge

**Sally Baxter MRCP FRCA**
Specialist Registrar in Anaesthesia and Intensive Care Medicine.
Wessex Deanery

**Andrew Breeze MA MRCOG**
Specialist Registrar in Obstetrics and Gynaecology
East of England Deanery

**Ash Chakraborty MS FRCS FRCR**
Consultant Paediatric Radiologist
Children's Hospital, Oxford

**Anita Chandra MSc MRCP DipRCPath**
Specialist Registrar, Department of Clinical Immunology
Addenbrooke's Hospital, Cambridge

**Anthony Edey MRCP FRCR**
Specialist Registrar in Clinical Radiology
King's College Hospital, London

**Nyree Griffin MD MRCS FRCR**
Consultant Radiologist
Guy's and St Thomas' Hospital, London

**Simon Milburn BSc MRCS FRCR**
Consultant Radiologist
James Cook Hospital, Middlesbrough

**Howard Portess MA FRCR**
Consultant Paediatric Radiologist
Southampton General Hospital

**Robin Proctor MA MRCP MRCGP**
Specialist Registrar in Clinical Radiology,
Wessex Deanery

**Evis Sala MD PhD FRCR**
Lecturer, Department of Radiology
University of Cambridge and Honorary Consultant Radiologist
Addenbrooke's Hospital, Cambridge

**Daniel Scoffings MRCP FRCR**
Consultant Neuroradiologist
Addenbrooke's Hospital
Cambridge University Hospitals NHS Trust

**Andrew Slater MRCP FRCR**
Consultant Radiologist
John Radcliffe Hospital, Oxford

**Edmund Soh BSc MRCP FRCR**
Associate Consultant Radiologist
Singapore General Hospital, Singapore.

**Dinuke R Warakaulle MRCP FRCR**
Consultant Interventional Radiologist
Stoke Mandeville Hospital, Aylesbury

# Introduction: approaches to emergency radiology

Richard Graham
Ferdia Gallagher

# How to use this book

*Emergencies in Radiology* is divided into two diagnostic sections.

There are a number of **introductory chapters** which help define the scope of emergency radiology and advise on writing relevant radiological reports. This is followed by a chapter on the 'real' radiological emergencies, such as cardiac arrest and contrast medium reactions, as well as how to manage them in the setting of a radiology department. The final introductory chapters review how best to care for patients within the radiology department in the emergency situation.

**The first diagnostic section** covers the common clinical presentations for each body region and suggests diagnostic algorithms for emergency radiology. It is divided into anatomical areas of the body rather than systems as, in our experience, emergency problems requiring imaging generally present to the radiologist in this way. For instance, a common request is for imaging in the context of acute abdominal pain: imaging of the abdomen is usually what the clinician asks for rather than imaging of the gastrointestinal tract. In addition, there is a final chapter in this section on post-operative imaging, which often requires different imaging strategies from those of a patient that has not recently undergone surgery.

We advise clinicians to use this section to aid their approach to imaging strategies and enable them to request the most helpful test that will reveal the diagnosis most quickly and with the least harm to the patient. Radiologists will also find this section useful if presented with a clinical problem that the clinician has not refined into a differential diagnosis as it can provide a logical imaging investigation strategy.

**The second diagnostic section** details specific conditions. It outlines the clinical and radiological findings in specific clinical entities which have been organized in a systems-based manner. There are two chapters in this section which are not systems-based: paediatric and interventional radiology. These have been included because their practice tends to be led by specialists in these disciplines alone. References to page numbers for interventional techniques have been included in the systems chapters.

This second section will be useful to those who face a defined clinical problem and are unsure on how or when to approach imaging. It will also be invaluable to those who are interpreting imaging investigations in the emergency setting: both radiologists and clinicians reviewing imaging of their patients.

In the second diagnostic section, a series of icons have been used to help indicate the level of urgency for imaging in each condition described. These can be found on the inside of the front cover.

# The role of the emergency radiologist

The provision of emergency radiology varies hugely between hospitals: some centres may have several consultants who specialize in emergency radiology while in many hospitals, a junior registrar may be primarily responsible for emergency imaging, especially out of hours. This book is aimed primarily at trainees in radiology and junior doctors in other specialties who refer patients for emergency imaging. The main aims of the book are to help all those involved in emergency radiological investigations to get the best and most appropriate use out of the radiology department and to provide patients requiring emergency imaging with the highest possible care.

# Thinking outside of the box

Patients are usually referred to the radiologist with a request to image a particular body area, e.g. the head, thorax etc. Unfortunately, such an approach can sometimes be unhelpful and misleading when trying to understand a patient's problem. *The role of the radiologist is to make a diagnosis rather than just to image the requested area.* It is not uncommon for the radiologist to be the most experienced doctor to review the case on-call and in such scenarios, the radiologist can help the referring clinician by 'thinking outside of the box'. For example: is the patient with abdominal pain having a myocardial infarct? Does the patient with profuse vomiting have a brain tumour? Does the patient with diaphragmatic irritation have appendicitis? Such diagnoses are not only immensely satisfying to make but may also save a patient's life.

## Further reading

**1.** Berrington de Gonzalez A and Darby S (2004) Risk of cancer from diagnostic X-rays: estimates for the UK and 14 other countries. *Lancet* **31**(363): 363–45.

# Emergency radiology as a subspecialty

The importance of emergency radiology has increased dramatically over the last decade in parallel with the rapid advancement of medical imaging. In the past, emergency radiology consisted largely of plain films interpreted by the referring clinician and re-reported by a radiologist at a later time when the result was often of academic interest only, as emergency management had been performed many hours or days before. Today, the radiologist is very much at the centre of emergency care and the outcome of medical imaging is central to patient management. Emergency radiology is not a subspecialty but rather the acute practice of all the main radiological subspecialties.

Emergency radiology can be defined as imaging that needs to be performed urgently in order to determine the best management of the patient. It needs to be differentiated from on-call radiology which is the subset of emergency radiology that occurs outside normal working hours and cannot wait until the next working day. For example, ultrasound (US) of the abdomen in a patient with classic symptoms of biliary colic and normal liver function tests (LFTs) is emergency radiology but would not be indicated out of hours. The result of the imaging test will not change management significantly overnight and no harm will come to the patient by waiting until the following morning for the US. Alternatively, a head computed tomography (CT) scan to exclude an extradural haematoma post head injury is quite different. This is an example of an investigation that needs to be performed urgently out of hours as it could alter acute management dramatically.

Currently, staffing levels on-call tend to be greatly reduced compared to a normal working day. The radiologist is often non-resident and is employed to provide only out of hours emergency radiology, not a routine emergency radiology service. Furthermore, if an interventional procedure is to be performed there is often only very limited support staff available and some centres do not make provision for this at all. This has a significant impact on the safety of on-call procedures.

We are in a period of transition in health care provision and as more resources are allocated to radiology, a 24hr 'routine' service may evolve. The *status quo* in most centres, however, is that imaging which will not change patient management is not usually performed out of hours.

# Emergency requests

## A brief guide for both clinicians and radiologists

Key points for any 'emergency' study are as follows:

- The most appropriate examination should be performed using the correct modality, i.e. US, CT, magnetic resonance imaging (MRI) etc.
- Imaging should be performed in an appropriate timescale. In particular, does this test need to be performed as an out of hours study?
- There should be a swift transfer of the results to the referring clinician for appropriate action to be instigated.
- Radiologists are *imaging doctors*, not technicians.

## Tips for the referring clinician

- **Clinical question.** Central to any radiological request should be the question that you wish answered. The clinical question may be critical in obtaining the correct answer: for instance a referral for a CT abdomen in a patient with right upper quadrant pain stating solely 'abdominal pain' may not reveal the true diagnosis. However, had the request stated all the relevant clinical details and asked if the patient had cholecystitis, the radiologist would usually have performed an ultrasound which is more sensitive and specific than CT for the disease and would not have exposed the patient to ionizing radiation. Inadequate clinical details on the request may therefore lead to inappropriate imaging which results in a delay in diagnosis and treatment.
- **Will the examination change management?** This is particularly pertinent to out of hours requests, as generally imaging investigations should only be performed if they will change the out of hours management of the patient.
- **Risk of the examination.** The clinician must always balance the potential risk of an examination with the potential benefits. Not only does the clinician have a responsibility to act in the best interest of the patient but they also have a legal responsibility when referring a patient for a study that involves ionizing radiation, i.e. X-ray, fluoroscopy, CT and nuclear medicine. Under the Ionizing Radiation (Medical Exposure) Regulations 2000 (IRMER), the referrer has a responsibility to provide sufficient medical information so that the radiologist can decide if the exposure can be justified.[1] Radiation risk is significant and 700 cases of cancer per year in the UK can be attributed to diagnostic radiation.[2] Radiation exposure is of particular importance if a woman is, or may be, pregnant and the referrer has a responsibility to inform the radiologist if this is the case. Even MRI has small potential risks: pacemakers are contraindicated and some implanted devices may be magnetic, e.g. prosthetic heart valves and aneurysm clips. In such cases it is best to find out the exact type of prosthesis before contacting the MRI department for advice. Metal workers may have small shards of metal within the orbit which can become dislodged during the study. Finally, all interventional procedures carry a small inherent risk which will be discussed in the appropriate chapters.

**What to put on the referral form.** Typically, referrals to radiology come in the form of paper or electronic requests. While there may be a temptation to exaggerate a patient's symptoms or signs to accelerate imaging, it may lead to an inappropriate test or even an unnecessary intervention.

**Include:** full patient name, hospital number, age or DOB, ward, means by which patient can travel to the department (e.g. chair), clinical history and your contact details. If your shift is about to finish then give the contact details of a colleague who will take action once the study has been reported and remember to contact them before leaving the hospital. Also include:

- History of **allergic reactions** to contrast medium.
- **Renal function:** elevated creatinine is associated with an increased risk of contrast medium induced nephropathy (📖 p. 24)
- **Pacemaker/metal prosthesis** for patients having an MRI.
- **Platelets** and **clotting** if the procedure involves intervention. If appropriate, consent the patient but only if you are suitably trained and qualified to do so.[3]
- **Pregnancy status** in women of reproductive age.
- **Infection risk,** e.g. MRSA.
- **Oxygen requirement** including flow rate.

- **What not to put on the referral form.** The decision to give intravenous (IV) contrast medium is generally made by the radiologist and there is no need to specify this on the form unless the patient has renal impairment and the clinical team is willing to dialyze the patient should acute renal failure result. It is best to ask a specific question rather than to ask for contrast medium to be given. For example, instead of asking for a CT with contrast medium, the clinician could ask if the hepatic artery is patent; in this case, an arterial study is necessary to answer the question but had the requester simply asked for a contrast-enhanced CT (CECT), a portal abdominal CT may have been performed and the question could have remained unanswered.

- **Contact the radiologist personally.** For any emergency study, it is of paramount importance that the referring doctor contacts the on-call radiologist personally and does not solely rely on an electronic referral system. Furthermore, a conversation with the radiologist may allow the complete clinical details to be discussed, thus ensuring that the patient has the appropriate examination in the appropriate timescale.

- **Who should refer a patient?** There is no simple answer to this question and different hospitals will have different policies. An experienced clinician should usually discuss a complicated case with an experienced radiologist. In general, the seniority of the referrer should be similar to that of the radiologist and in all cases it should be someone who knows the full clinical details.

- **Patient escort.** Once a study has been agreed and a time arranged, remember to inform the ward. Most hospitals will insist that an unwell patient is escorted to the radiology department with a nurse but occasionally they may also require a doctor, e.g. anaesthetist.

- **Reviewing the report.** The referrer bears the responsibility of checking the radiologist's report and acting accordingly. In the case of unexpected or immediately life-threatening findings, the radiologist should also contact the referring clinician directly.[4]

## Tips for the emergency radiologist

- **Always be contactable**. Make sure the hospital switchboard has an up to date list of who is on call and that they have your full contact details. As rota changes occur frequently, it may be appropriate at the beginning of an on-call to ring the switchboard and check that they know your preferred method of contact.

- **Polite but firm**. While there may be good reasons for being irritated by a poor-quality referral, being rude to a clinician is not constructive or helpful.

- **Clinical disagreements and acting in the best interests of the patient**. The on-call radiologist must not perform a test that they feel is inappropriate, unnecessary or puts the patient at unwanted risk (e.g. radiation risk as controlled by IRMER). If, after discussion, the referring clinician still feels it is appropriate to perform a test that the on-call radiologist disagrees with, then further advice should be sought. If a junior clinician has requested an examination that is under discussion, it is reasonable for the radiologist to ask to speak with the most senior doctor caring for the patient. Most misunderstandings are resolved at this stage but very occasionally a disagreement will persist, and in such cases a consultant-to-consultant discussion should occur. However, in all circumstances, the *patient's best interest must be paramount* and local guidelines/departmental policy should be adhered to.

- **Accept responsibility for the patient**. Sometimes a clinician may be given differing opinions by several radiologists on a particular case, e.g. regarding which imaging modality to use first. While these differing opinions may all be valid, such a scenario is clearly frustrating to the referrer. It is the authors' opinion that when a patient is referred to a radiologist, they should take responsibility for arranging the required imaging for that patient. This may take many forms, e.g. actually performing the study, speaking with the appropriate radiologist, leaving a message for someone else in the department, or even nothing if the test will be done in a timely fashion during normal working hours. The important point is that the radiologist receiving the request has taken responsibility for ensuring that the correct study will be performed in an appropriate timescale.

- **Patient details**. When accepting a referral, it is important to take all the necessary details described above. A patient escort is particularly important when working alone in the department as it may be difficult to call for help if the patient's condition deteriorates. If the clinician is to end their shift shortly, then it is important to get the contact details of someone who will be caring for the patient when the test has been performed.

- **Contacting the clinician with the results.** Hospital policies differ but generally it is appropriate to contact the clinician with the results of an on-call study. Although it is ultimately the responsibility of a clinician to check a report, when an immediately life-threatening abnormality is detected the radiologist should bring this to the attention of the clinician as rapidly as possible via direct telephone communication.[4]

## Further reading

**1.** Department of Health (2000) *Ionising Radiation (Medical Exposure) Regulations 2000*. HMSO, London, UK.

**2.** Berrington de Gonzalez A and Darby S (2004) Risk of cancer from diagnostic X-rays. *Lancet* **31**(363); 363–45.

**3.** Royal College of Radiologists (2005) *Standards for Patient Consent Particular to Radiology*. Royal College of Radiologists, London.

**4.** Royal College of Radiologists (2006) *Standards for the Reporting and Interpretation of Imaging Investigations*. Royal College of Radiologists, London.

# The role of the trainee in emergency radiology

The radiologist provides the continuum between the patient, the referring clinician and the sequence of radiological investigations.

RCR guidelines suggest that trainees should be working on an on-call rota during the third year of training if not before.[1] While on-calls may appear daunting at first, preparation can make them less frightening and more rewarding:

- Ask a more experienced trainee for tips on how to best approach on-calls in your hospital(s). Even simple things such as knowing where the on-call bleep is kept can reduce stress.
- Find out what your local hospital guidelines are, what you are expected to do out of hours and what you are not.
- Before you start your first on-call, make sure you are confident in the basic interpretation of the imaging you are likely to encounter as outlined in this book.

Always remember that the trainee is just that: *a trainee*. You are not expected to know all the answers and indeed even experienced consultants refer to other colleagues for help with a difficult case. Consultant radiologists have been shown to have a clinically significant discrepancy rate in their reporting of head CTs of ~2 % (when compared to neuro-radiologists.[2]) Furthermore, trainees have been shown to be more likely to overcall abnormalities on trauma radiographs than consultant radiologists.[3] *Asking for help should not be considered a sign of failure or weakness and should never be treated as such.* RCR guidelines state that on-calls should be performed with 'appropriate consultant back-up'.[1] Clearly this support varies depending on the trainee's level of experience but it should always be readily available when requested.

## Misses, misinterpretations and other errors

Follow-up is an essential element of personal education. Working in a vacuum on-call is not only of poor educational value but can be dangerous. After all, if we do not realize that we are making the same errors then we will continue to make them. As a trainee there are numerous approaches that can be taken to minimize errors:

- Ask the consultant on-call to review your reports. If the answer to the question would change management of the patient out of hours then the consultant should be called immediately. Teleradiology will make reviewing images at home increasingly feasible. However, if the problem is not critical, the images can be reviewed the following morning. It is important to contact the clinicians if any significant changes have been made to a provisional report following this review.
- Find out the definitive diagnosis. This may be determined from later radiological tests, blood tests, from pathological specimens, at the time of surgery or at post-mortem. Contacting the clinician the next day may be enlightening.
- Personal audit. Keeping a record of all the patients you have imaged on-call will allow the trainee to audit their performance.

- Feedback to your colleagues. This is important if you find others have made mistakes and a 'no-blame' culture is essential for a healthy learning environment.
- Attending discrepancy/errors meetings. Learning from the mistakes of others may help you avoid making the same error yourself.
- Attending multidisciplinary team (MDT) meetings. Most interesting cases are reviewed at one or more MDT. These allow the opportunity for a second opinion to be given as well as comparing the radiological results with other non-imaging tests.
- The dangers of 'overcalling'. There is often a common perception that 'overcalling' a suspected abnormality as abnormal is better than 'undercalling' it by suggesting it may be a normal variant. While this may usually be the case, this approach underestimates the financial and human cost of unnecessary and potentially invasive further tests and treatment. Radiology is driven by experience—generally the more you have seen the better you are. *Asking for a second opinion from a more experienced radiologist should never be undervalued.*

## Further reading

**1.** Royal College of Radiologists (2007) *Structured Training Curriculum for Clinical Radiology*. Royal College of Radiologists. http://www.rcr.ac.uk/docs/radiology/pdf/Curriculum-CR-Jan2007.pdf

**2.** Erly WK, Boyd C, Lucio RW *et al.* (2003) Evaluation of emergency CT scans of the head: is there a common standard? *AJR* **180**; 1727–30.

**3.** Williams SM, Connelly DJ, Wadsworth S *et al.* (2000) Radiological review of accident and emergency radiographs. *Clin Rad* **55**; 861–5.

# Writing reports and radiological terminology

## Report writing

The art of writing reports is tailoring them to the referring clinician, answering the clinical question and stating important negatives that are implicit from the request. Reports should not be too long—otherwise the clinicians will probably not read them—or too short, e.g. normal abdominal appearances, as the clinician may want to know whether you remembered to look at the bones.

### Suggested layout

- Indication: A precis of the clinical information, including any clinical questions to be answered.
- Technique: A short description of the technique used stating weather contrast was used. If MRI, then the sequences should be recorded. The anatomical region imaged should also be recorded.
- Findings: A sentence regarding the technical adequacy of the study and any limitations. A concise description of the important positive and negative findings. Two common styles are numbered points or paragraphs of text.
- Conclusion: This should contain the answer to a clinical question that has been posed. Furthermore, the most important findings should be highlighted, including unexpected findings and any suggestions for further imaging/management included.

# Radiological terminology

A full description of radiological terminology is beyond the scope of this book but is it is important to use the appropriate term when describing the appearance of images from each of the major radiological modalities. The following may be helpful to non-radiologists in understanding the radiological report:

**Radiographs** Radio-opacity or density: radio-opaque is white or bright and radiolucent is black or dark.
**Ultrasound** Echogenicity or reflectivity: ↑echogenicity is white or bright.
**CT** Density or Hounsfield Units (HU): ↑density is white or bright with a high HU value.
**MRI** Signal: ↑Signal is white or bright.

# Emergencies in radiology

## ☠ Adult Basic Life Support (BLS) and in-hospital resuscitation

### Definition
Maintenance of an adequate circulation and ventilation until action can be taken to treat the underlying cause of the cardiopulmonary arrest. The division between basic and advanced life support following an in-hospital cardiac arrest is arbitrary, the process being a continuum.

### Clinical features
- Patient collapsed and unresponsive.
- Cardiopulmonary arrest may be due to a primary airway, breathing or cardiovascular problem.

### Immediate management for the collapsed patient in hospital

*See In-hospital Resuscitation Algorithm,* 📖 *p16*
- Ensure it is safe to approach the patient, e.g. stop screening/scanning. May need to remove the patient from scanner to enable assessment.

#### Check patient for a response:
- Gently shake patient's shoulders and ask loudly "Are you alright?" (Do not shake shoulders if cervical spine injury suspected.)

#### If patient responds:
- Assess using the **A**irway, **B**reathing, **C**irculation, **D**isability and **E**xposure approach and begin basic treatment, e.g. oxygen, monitoring, IV access.
- Call for further help as required, e.g. resuscitation or medical emergency team.

#### If patient does not respond:
- Shout for help.
- Open airway by tilting head and lifting chin (if suspected cervical spine injury avoid head tilt. Use chin lift/jaw thrust).
- Look in mouth and remove visible foreign body/debris.
- Keeping airway open, look, listen and feel for breathing for a maximum of 10s. Agonal breathing (infrequent, noisy gasps) is a sign of cardiac arrest.
- Simultaneously check for signs of movement/life/pulse.

#### If the patient has a pulse or signs of life:
- Assess patient using ABCDE and call for help as required.

## If there is no pulse or signs of life (cardiac arrest):
- Start cardiopulmonary resuscitation (CPR).
  - Send others to call the cardiac arrest team and collect resuscitation equipment. If alone leave patient briefly to call arrest team. Start CPR on returning.
  - If in MRI remove patient from scan room on a non-magnetic trolley to outside the 0.5mT boundary. Most resuscitation equipment cannot enter the MRI scan room.
- Give 30 compressions followed by 2 ventilations (same ratios for 1 or 2 rescuers).
  - Compressions: place hands in centre of lower half of sternum. Depth of compressions: 4–5 cm. Rate: 100/min. Allow chest to fully recoil between compressions. Minimize interruptions in compressions.
  - Ventilations: maintain airway and ventilate (use available equipment, e.g. pocket mask or bag and mask with oral airway). Use inspiratory time of 1s and enough volume to produce a chest rise similar to normal breathing. Watch chest fall between ventilations. Add supplemental oxygen as soon as possible.
- Continue CPR 30:2— a ratio of 30 chest compression to 2 breaths— until patient is intubated, then change to uninterrupted chest compressions at rate of 100/min and simultaneous ventilation at rate of 10/min.
- As soon as defibrillator arrives attach electrodes and check rhythm. Defibrillate if appropriate and trained to do so (follow voice prompts if using automated external defibrillator [AED]).
- Recommence CPR immediately after defibrillation.
- Obtain IV access as soon as possible.
- Change person providing chest compressions every 2mins to prevent fatigue.
- Continue resuscitation until resuscitation team arrives or patient shows signs of life.

## If the patient is not breathing but has a pulse (respiratory arrest):
- Ventilate the patient (as above) rechecking the pulse every 10 breaths. If there is any doubt about the presence of a pulse treat as a cardiac arrest.

## Subsequent management
- If resuscitation is successful the patient will require transfer to a suitable high care area in the hospital.

## Further reading
UK Resuscitation Council Guidelines (2005) http://www.resus.org.uk/pages/guide.htm

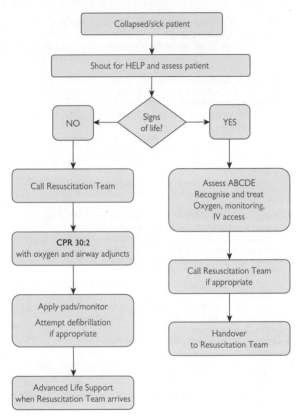

**Fig. 2.1** Adult In-hospital Resuscitation Algorithm.[1]

1. With permission of the Resuscitation Council, UK.

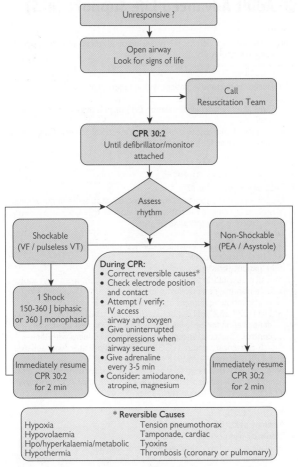

**Fig. 2.2** Adult Advanced Life Support Algorithm.[1]

---

**1.** With permission of the Resuscitation Council, UK.

## ☢ Adult Advanced Life Support (ALS)

### Definition
- A structured approach for the provision of advanced skills to support vital organ function.

### Presentation
- Collapsed, unresponsive patient with no signs of life.
- Cardiac rhythm may be:
  - Shockable: ventricular fibrillation (VF) or pulseless ventricular tachycardia (VT).
  - Non-shockable: asystole or pulseless electrical activity (PEA). This is more common for in hospital cardiac arrests.

### Immediate management
📖 *ALS algorithm,* 📖 *p.17*
- Ensure it is safe to approach the patient, e.g. stop screening/scanning. May need to remove the patient from scanner to enable assessment.
- If the patient is unresponsive:
  - Shout for help.
  - Open the airway (remember cervical spine).
  - Check for signs of life.
- If the patient shows no signs of life:
  - Call resuscitation team. If in MRI remove patient from scan room on a non-magnetic trolley to beyond the 0.5mT boundary. Most resuscitation equipment can not enter the MRI scan room.
  - Start CPR 30:2 until defibrillator/monitor attached. Do not delay defibrillation for basic life support (BLS), IV access or airway control. Chance of successful defibrillation reduces with time.
- Attach electrocardiogram (ECG) monitor/defibrillator (without stopping CPR).
- Assess rhythm (will need to stop CPR briefly due to interference of compressions) and decide if VF/pulseless VT i.e. shockable or non-VF/VT (PEA/asystole) i.e. non-shockable.

### If VF/pulseless VT:
- Attempt defibrillation.
- Paddle or pad position:
  - Place one below right clavicle in mid-clavicular line.
  - Place second in the left mid-axillary line approximately level with V6 ECG electrode or female breast.
  - Many defibrillators are now hands free. If using manual paddles remember to use gel pads and press paddles firmly onto chest. Only charge defibrillator when paddles are in contact with patient.
  - Either paddle/pad can be placed in either position.
- Oxygen masks, nasal cannulae or ventilation bags should be removed during defibrillation and placed at least 1m away from patient's chest.

# ☣ Adverse reactions to contrast media

Adverse reactions to intravenous contrast media can be classified as either general or organ-specific.

The general reactions can be further divided into acute or delayed: delayed adverse reactions predominantly affect the skin and occur 1 hour to 1 week after injection.

Although there are numerous organ-specific reactions, e.g. cardiovascular, pulmonary and neurological, the most common are extravasation of contrast medium and contrast-induced nephrotoxicity, both of which will be considered here.

Finally, the special cases of pregnancy and lactation will be discussed.

## Clinical features of a contrast medium reaction

- **Mild reactions**: nausea, vomiting, mild urticaria (raised, itchy and erythematous wheals or 'hives'), pallor and pain in the injected extremity. These are usually short in duration and self-limiting. Generally they do not require specific treatment.
- **Moderate reactions**: severe vomiting, extensive urticaria, laryngeal angioedema, dyspnoea and rigors.
- **Severe reactions**: pulmonary oedema, cardiac arrhythmias, cardiac arrest, circulatory collapse, and unconsciousness.

Moderate and severe reactions require immediate management.

## Practical safety considerations for the radiologist

- A doctor should always be immediately available to manage any adverse reaction. However, this does not have to be a radiologist.
- All radiologists should familiarize themselves with the basic management of contrast medium reactions as well as where the appropriate drugs are stored in the department.
- In the presence of risk factors, the decision about contrast media administration should be taken by the radiologist supervising the procedure. Intravascular iodinated contrast medium should not be administered if the patient is hyperthyroid.[1] Avoid giving iodinated contrast medium in pregnancy where possible.[1]
- Facilities for management of adverse reactions should be clearly visible, easy to obtain and regularly checked.
- A patient should be monitored for the first 5min and should remain on the premises for at least 15–20min after injection. The majority of severe reactions occur within this time.
- All contrast media reactions should be formally documented with details of their nature, severity and the agent used.

# Acute general reactions

## Aetiology and epidemiology

The risk of a mild adverse reaction is fivefold lower with non-ionic rather than ionic contrast media and tenfold lower for severe reactions. Severe reactions occur in 0.04% of patients who receive non-ionic contrast media. Fatal reactions are rare: 1:170 000.[2]

Recurrent adverse reactions occur in 17–35% of patients with a history of a previous adverse reaction to ionic contrast media. Recurrent adverse events are much lower with non-ionic contrast media occurring in 5%.

There are several predisposing risk factors to these reactions (see box below) and all patients must be evaluated for risk factors prior to injection with contrast media. In the presence of risk factors, the need for contrast medium should be re-evaluated: for instance an initial unenhanced CT study could be performed before making the decision to give contrast medium and other potential methods of investigation should be considered, e.g. US.

> ## Predisposing risk factors for general acute reactions to contrast media
> - Infants and the elderly:
>   - Reactions are more severe in the elderly
> - History of previous reaction to contrast media:
>   - Risk of a severe reaction ↑fivefold
> - History of allergy:
>   - Increases risk threefold
>   - There is no specific cross-reactivity with shellfish or topical iodine in acute reactions
> - History of asthma:
>   - Tenfold ↑risk for high osmolality contrast media
>   - Sixfold ↑for low osmolality contrast media
> - Dehydration
> - Heart disease
> - Pre-existing renal disease
> - Haematological conditions:
>   - e.g. sickle cell disease, polycythaemia, and myeloma
> - Drugs:
>   - Beta-blockers, non-steroidal anti-inflammatory drugs (NSAIDs) and interleukin-2

## Treatment in adults

- **Mild reactions**: retain IV access and observe the patient until fully recovered. Pruritus/urticaria can be treated with chlorphenamine maleate 4–8 mg *per os* (PO) or with a non-sedating antihistamine, e.g cetirizine 10 mg PO.
- **Moderate reactions**: chlorphenamine 10–20mg IV over 2min for severe urticaria. Moderate wheeze may be treated with 100% $O_2$ inhalation (10–15L/min) and nebulized salbutamol (5mg in 2ml saline).
- **Severe reactions**: see box below. Also see BLS/ALS chapter: 📖 p. 17.

## Treatment of severe general acute adverse reactions to contrast in adults

**Laryngeal angioedema**
- Oxygen by mask (6–10 L/min)
- Adrenaline (1:1000) 0.5 ml IM injection

**Severe bronchospasm**
- Oxygen by mask (6–10L/min)
- Nebulized salbutamol (5 mg in 2 ml saline)
- Adrenaline injection if bronchospasm is progressive

**Hypotension without bradycardia**
- Elevate patient's legs
- Oxygen by mask (6–10L/min)
- Intravenous fluids (normal saline or Ringer's lactate)
- If unresponsive: give adrenaline (1:1000) 0.5 ml IM injection and repeat as needed; see also BLS/ALS chapters 📖 p. 17.

**Vagal reaction**
- Elevate patient's legs
- Oxygen by mask (6–10L/min)
- Intravenous fluids (normal saline or Ringer's lactate)
- Atropine 0.3mg IV; repeat if necessary every 3–5min up to 3mg in total.

**Generalised anaphylactoid reaction**: treatment acronym, **COOLFAST**

| | |
|---|---|
| C | Call for resuscitation team |
| O | Open airways |
| O | Oxygen by mask (6–10L/min) |
| L | Leg elevation |
| F | Fluids IV (normal saline or Ringer's lactate) |
| A | Adrenaline (1:1000) 0.5ml (0.5mg) IM injection with ECG monitoring |
| ST | Steroids: hydrocortisone 200mg IM or slow IV and 10mg chlorphenamine IM or slow IV |

## Prevention

Various treatment regimens for the prevention of adverse reactions to contrast media have been proposed and include corticosteroids ± anti-histamines. Specific individual advice for each patient should be obtained from the local clinical immunology or allergy service.

# Delayed general reactions

These are more common in young adults, women and patients with a history of allergy. There is a higher incidence with the use of iso-osmolar non-ionic contrast media. Most reactions are mild to moderate and self-limiting. Symptoms include mild urticaria and angioedema. Prophylaxis is not generally recommended.

# Extravasation of IV contrast medium

Intravenous contrast medium extravasation occurs in 0.035–0.2% of patients with the use of mechanical power injectors. Clinical presentation includes burning pain, tenderness, oedema and erythema. Severe injury results in blistering, sloughing of skin and compartment syndrome. Initial treatment is elevation of the affected extremity, ice packs and close observation for 2–4 hours. Plastic surgery consultation is recommended if the injected volume of non-ionic contrast media exceeds 100ml (30ml if ionic).

# Contrast-induced nephrotoxicity

- Contrast-induced nephrotoxicity is defined as an increase in baseline serum creatinine of at least 44µmol/L (0.5mg/dl) within 48 hours of injection of the contrast.
- The risk of nephrotoxicity is increased to 12–27% in the presence of pre-existing renal impairment (especially diabetic nephropathy), with the risk being related to the extent of pre-existing renal impairment, the dose of contrast media administered and the state of hydration of the patient. For this group of patients, non-ionic contrast medium is less nephrotoxic than ionic agents.
- Other risk factors include: heart failure, hyperuricaemia, old age, large dose of contrast and concomitant use of other nephrotoxic drugs.
- All patients with renal impairment, especially diabetics, should have serum creatinine measured prior to administration of contrast medium. Royal College of Radiologists (RCR) guidelines suggest a level of 130 µmol/L indicates renal impairment. Measurement of the glomerular filtration rate (GFR) is a more sensitive indicator of renal impairment and is recommended for high-risk patients. If the use of contrast media is unavoidable, then ensure that the patient is adequately hydrated and use the smallest dose possible of low osmolar non-ionic monomeric or iso-osmolar non-ionic dimeric contrast medium.
- ☛The prophylactic use of N-acetylcysteine and sodium bicarbonate has been suggested to prevent contrast-induced nephropathy in high-risk patients but their use is controversial.
- Patients taking metformin are at risk of lactic acidosis, which may be fatal, if renal excretion of the drug if reduced. This can be exacerbated by the addition of IV contrast. Even if the serum creatinine is normal, when more than 100mls of contrast media is administered then metformin should be withheld for 48hrs after the injection. In the presence of renal impairment and when contrast media is unavoidable,

metformin should be withheld for 48hrs pre- and post-procedure. Alternative diabetic control with insulin may need to be instigated. Renal function should be reassessed prior to recommencing metformin.
• In the emergency situation IV contrast medium may have to be given to a patient with renal failure who is on metformin, as the benefits to the patient of imaging outweigh the risk of lactic acidosis. In this situation, the clinician must be made aware and must withhold the metformin and check the renal function for 48 hours post-procedure.

# Pregnancy and breastfeeding

Iodinated contrast media can cross the human placenta; therefore, unless there is an exceptional reason, the use of contrast media is contraindicated. If it has to be administered then thyroid function in the neonate should be measured in the first week after birth because of the theoretical risk of thyroid suppression.[1]

Only a very small amount of iodinated contrast medium passes into the breast milk and virtually none of this is absorbed by the baby. Therefore, no special precaution is required for breastfeeding.[1]

## Further reading

**1.** Board of the Faculty of Clinical Radiology, RCR (2005) *Standards for Iodinated Intravascular Contrast Agent Administration to Adult Patients.* Available at http://www.rcr.ac.uk/docs/radiology/pdf/IVcontrastPrintFinal.pdf.

**2.** Namasivayam S, Kalra MK, Torres WE *et al.* (2006) Adverse reactions to intravenous iodinated contrast media: a primer for radiologists. *Emerg Radiol* **12**; 210–15.

**3.** Namasivayam S, Kalra MK, Torres WE *et al.* (2006) Adverse reactions to intravenous iodinated contrast media: an update. *Curr Probl Diag Radiol* **35**; 164–9.

# Patient care in radiology

# Patient management prior to imaging

### General principles
- Patients should be appropriately resuscitated and stabilized by the referring teams prior to transfer to the radiology department whenever possible (Imaging the unstable patient 📖 p. 30).

### Patients with a decreased level of consciousness
- Patients with a Glasgow Coma Score (GCS) of ≤8 should be discussed with the on-call anaesthetist as intubation for imaging (usually CT head) may be appropriate. *This can take some time to organize.*
- Some patients may be more safely imaged in the recovery position.

### Glasgow Coma Score
- Best motor response:
  - 6 – Obeys verbal commands
  - 5 – Localizes to pain
  - 4 – Withdraws from pain
  - 3 – Flexion to pain
  - 2 – Extension to pain
  - 1 – No response
- Best eye opening response:
  - 4 – Eyes spontaneously open
  - 3 – Eyes open to command
  - 2 – Eyes open in response to pain
  - 1 – No response
- Best verbal response:
  - 5 – Fully orientated
  - 4 – Confused
  - 3 – Inappropriate words
  - 2 – Incomprehensible sounds
  - 1 – No response

### If planned investigation requires IV contrast (See 📖 p. 24)
- Use of IV contrast carries the potential risk of nephrotoxicity.

# Imaging the unstable patient

## General principles

- The radiology department is a potentially dangerous place for the unstable patient due to limited equipment and staffing, the often remote nature of the department and the limited access to the patient during imaging.
- Portable imaging at the bedside may be a safer option (the images obtained, although suboptimal, may be sufficient to answer the clinical question).
- Ensure that the scan is appropriate and that it is not delaying definitive treatment unnecessarily.
- Unstable patients should be accompanied by a suitably trained doctor. They should be monitored throughout transfer to and from the radiology department and during the imaging itself and will require ongoing oxygen therapy.
- Transferring unstable and/or ventilated patients to the radiology department can be difficult and requires a lot of specialist equipment (monitors, ventilators, oxygen cylinders, syringe pumps, defibrillators, and drugs, etc.) to travel with the patient.
- Due to the condition of the patient and the equipment required unexpected delays in leaving the ward area for imaging are sometimes unavoidable.
- Minimize the time the unstable patient needs to spend within the department.

## Pre imaging

- Assess the risks and benefits of imaging each unstable patient individually.
- Ensure the referring team understand what the imaging entails, if it is likely to be tolerated (e.g. a patient with respiratory distress may be unable to lie flat) and the likely yield from the investigation.
- Patients should be stabilized prior to transfer to the radiology department whenever possible. This may not be possible when the patient is coming for radiological intervention, e.g. embolization.
- Patients with a GCS of 8 or less should be discussed with an anaesthetist. Such patients may require intubating prior to imaging and/or be accompanied by an anaesthetist.
- Check that long oxygen tubing is available to reach the patient when positioned for scanning.
- Ensure adequate venous access prior to imaging–particularly if contrast or interventional procedures are planned. Remote injection ports can be useful especially if the patient is draped. Remember to flush through any drugs.
- Unstable patients often have deranged renal function. Potential risks/ benefits of using contrast should be considered on an individual basis (Patient management prior to imaging 🕮 p. 24).

## During imaging

- Ensure adequate monitoring (e.g. pulse oximetry, blood pressure, ECG) and continuous oxygen therapy.

- Check that lines, oxygen/ventilator tubing, drains and catheters are all suitably positioned to allow free and safe movement of the patient and scanner.
- Monitoring and ongoing treatment of the patient should be undertaken by a separate member of staff—not the radiologist.
- Some patients will need to be accompanied in the scan room by a suitably trained member of staff throughout the imaging. Advise them of the safest place to stand.
- Optimum positioning and breath holding may not be possible. Keep patients with respiratory problems sat up for as much time as possible.
- Scans may have to be abandoned or interrupted if the patient's condition deteriorates.

Post imaging

- Imaging results should be made available to the referring team as soon as possible.
- Advise referring team of any ongoing radiology issues, e.g. drains *in situ*, further imaging requirements, use of contrast and need to monitor renal function (especially in diabetics taking metformin).

# Sedation and analgesia

Sedation and analgesia can make unpleasant procedures safer and more acceptable to patients but they have the potential to cause life-threatening complications.

## Definitions

- Sedation is 'a technique in which the use of a drug or drugs produces a state of depression of the central nervous system enabling treatment to be carried out, but during which verbal contact with the patient is maintained throughout the period of sedation'.[1]
- Analgesia is the suppression of pain from a normally painful stimulus.
- Pain is an unpleasant sensory and emotional experience resulting from a stimulus causing, or likely to cause, tissue damage.

## General principles

- Patient safety is paramount.
- Sympathetic patient management with clear explanations may allay anxiety and reduce the need for sedation and analgesia.
- Intravenous sedatives and opioids cause respiratory depression, particularly when used in combination.
- Analgesics should be given before sedatives to reduce the risk of respiratory suppression.
- All doses should be given incrementally and the minimum dose used so the patient remains rousable.
- Extra caution is required in the frail and elderly:
  - Use smaller initial doses and increments.
  - Allow longer between increments—low cardiac output and a slow arm—brain circulation time delays onset of effect.
  - Beware of co-morbidities and adjust maximum doses.
  - Check patient's weight if they appear particularly small.
- Check if patients have already received sedatives or potent analgesics, e.g. given in A&E, and reduce doses accordingly.
- Use local anaesthesia for all percutaneous techniques regardless of sedation and analgesia.

## Analgesia

- Simple analgesics (NSAIDs and paracetamol) may be given pre-procedure and can reduce the amount of opioid required. They may also help patients who have joint problems to lie still in comfort.
- Opioid analgesics may be required for interventional procedures. Non-vascular procedures (especially renal and hepatobiliary) tend to be more painful than vascular ones.
- Consider opioid patient-controlled analgesia for post procedural pain.
- Entonox may be useful for short, painful procedures.

## Commonly used analgesics (adults)

- Opioids
  - Also have some sedative effects.
  - Side-effects include: respiratory depression, drowsiness, nausea and vomiting, constipation, hypotension and ureteric and biliary spasm.
  - Fentanyl is approximately a 50–80 times more potent analgesic than morphine and is more rapidly titratable.

|  | Morphine | Fentanyl |
|---|---|---|
| Presentation | Syrup, tablets, suppositories and solution for injection (1mg/ml minijets or ampoules of 10, 15, 20, 30mg/ml). | Lozenges, transdermal patches and solution for injection (50mcg/ml). |
| IV dose | Total 0.1–0.15mg/kg. Generally titrated as 1–2mg boluses every 5min. Usual total dose 2–10mg. Often used as PCA e.g. 1mg bolus with 5min lockout. | Total 1–5mcg/kg. Generally 50–100mcg initial bolus followed by increments of 25–50mcg every 2–5min. Caution at doses greater than 200mcg. |
| Onset of effect | Slow onset IV, peak effect 15–20min. | Rapid onset of action IV, peak effect 2–5min. |
| Duration of effect | Long acting, lasts 3–4hrs IV | Short acting, lasts 30–60min IV. |

- Entonox
  - Ready-mixed cylinders of a 50/50 mixture of nitrous oxide and oxygen.
  - Usually self-administered with a demand valve.
  - Both sedative and analgesic effect
  - Rapid onset and short recovery time.
  - May cause nausea and vomiting.
  - Contraindicated in patients with pneumothorax. Use with caution in conditions with closed air containing spaces, e.g. intestinal obstruction, bullos lung disease.

## Local and regional anaesthesia

- Use local anaesthesia for all percutaneous techniques regardless of sedation and analgesia (may also be useful under general anaesthesia).
- Topical local anaesthetic creams can be used to make venepuncture more tolerable in needle-phobics.
- Some procedures may benefit from regional anaesthetic techniques, e.g. interpleural or paraspinal blocks.
- When estimating the safe dosage consider patient age, weight, physique, clinical condition, rate of absorption and excretion. More vascular areas absorb local anaesthetic faster than less vascular areas which may cause a higher peak concentration.
- Inadvertent intravascular injection of local anaesthetics is potentially life-threatening.

## Commonly used local anaesthetics

- (1% solution contains 10mg/ml, 0.5% solution contains 5g/ml etc.)
- Lidocaine (lignocaine)
  - Available as 0.5%, 1%, 2% solution for injection (4% and 5% as spray or topical ointment).
  - Maximum dose 3mg/kg/4hrs (Increased to 7mg/kg/4hrs with adrenaline 1 in 200 000 (5mcg/ml)). Do not use adrenaline in digits and appendages.
- Bupivacaine
  - Available as 0.25% and 0.5% solution for injection.
  - Maximum dose 2mg/kg/4hrs (dose not increased by co-administration of adrenaline).
  - Levobupivacaine (an isomer of bupivacaine) may have fewer adverse effects. Same dose as bupivacaine.
- Topical creams (Apply topically under an occlusive dressing)
  - EMLA (lignocaine 2.5% with prilocaine 2.5%). Local anaesthesia within 1–2hrs for up to 5hrs. Avoid in children less than 1 year of age.
  - Ametop (amethocaine 4%). Local anaesthesia within 30–45min for up to 4hrs. Licensed for use on children over 4 weeks of age.

## Local anaesthetic toxicity

- Symptoms and signs:
  - Tingling (typically around mouth and tongue)
  - Light-headedness, agitation and tremor
  - Convulsions and/or unconsciousness
  - Cardiovascular collapse. Hypotension may be cased by hypox-aemia due to central apnoea, direct myocardial suppression or vasodilatation. Arrhythmias may occur (resistant ventricular arrhythmias are more likely with bupivacaine).
- Treatment:
  - Stop injection/administration
  - Supportive: ABCDE with oxygen, seizure control and cardiovas-cular support.
  - Some evidence for the use of IV Intralipid® in treatment of local anaesthetic-induced cardiac arrest.[2]

## Sedation

- May be oral, intranasal (most common in paediatrics) or intravenous.
- Verbal contact and a response to non-painful physical stimuli must be maintained at all times, otherwise the patient is anaesthetised.

## Commonly used intravenous sedatives (adults)

- Midazolam
  - Benzodiazepine.
  - No analgesic effect.
  - Sedative effects may be unpredictable. Can cause paradoxical agitation in higher doses.
  - Amnesic effect greater than sedative effect.
  - Narrow safety margin. Respiratory depression in higher doses or on rapid injection.
  - Presentation: solution for injection 1mg/ml, 2mg/ml or 5mg/ml.
  - Dose IV: initially 2–2.5mg (0.5–1mg in elderly), increased if necessary after 2min in 1mg (0.5mg in elderly) steps every 2min. Usual total dose 3.5–5mg.
  - Duration of effect: 30min–2hrs.
- Diazepam
  - Benzodiazepine.
  - No longer recommended as it is thrombogenic IV and has a long duration of action.

### Pre-procedure

- Patients receiving intravenous sedation must be starved as if having a general anaesthetic.
  - 6hrs for food and milk (including milk in tea and coffee)
  - 2hrs for clear fluids e.g. water, black tea or coffee.
- Consent for procedures requiring sedation/analgesia should be obtained prior to the patient arriving in the radiology department. This may not be possible in the emergency setting.

### Safety during sedation and analgesia

- Only give intravenous sedation/analgesia if competent to do so.
- Use drugs that you are familiar with.
- Ensure all syringes are clearly labelled with drug name and concentration. Consider using internationally standardized colour-coded labels and different sized syringes for different drugs.
- Speak to an anaesthetist if you are concerned.
- Obtain secure intravenous access.
- Oxygen:
  - Give oxygen to all patients receiving intravenous sedation/analgesia (e.g. start with nasal cannulae or face mask at 2–4L/min and increase if required).
  - Start before the first dose of sedative/analgesic and continue throughout the procedure and recovery.
  - Monitor oxygen saturation ($SpO_2$) continuously.
  - Aim to keep $SpO_2$ at or above 95%.
  - A $SpO_2$ below 90% is dangerous and requires immediate intervention (ABCDE approach).
- Monitoring:
  - A suitably trained assistant must monitor the patient throughout the duration of the sedation/analgesia. This may involve staying in the

scan room itself during screening. The radiologist performing the procedure can NOT monitor the level of sedation adequately.

- Watch the patient and respond to evidence of pain. Consider additional analgesia if simpler methods such as reassurance, hand-holding, etc. are insufficient.
- Continuous pulse oximetry is mandatory. Other monitoring may be appropriate, e.g. blood pressure (BP, automated), respiratory rate, ECG.
- Observations should be recorded.
- Specially compatible monitors are required for MRI. Put padding between patient's skin and cables and avoid loops of cable which can induce current and burns.
- Other equipment:
  - Full resuscitation equipment and reversal agents readily available. See Table 3.1.
  - Patients should be managed on a tipping trolley with suction readily available wherever possible (if patient vomits whilst sedated, turn them into the lateral position, tilt trolley head down to minimize risk of aspiration. Use suction to remove obvious vomit).

**Table 3.1** Reversal agents

|  | Naloxone | Flumazenil |
|---|---|---|
| **Antagonises** | Opioids | Benzodiazepines |
| **Presentation** | Clear colourless solution: 400mcg/ml or 1mg/ml | Clear colourless solution: 100mcg/ml |
| **Initial IV dose** | 0.4–2mg (paediatrics: 10mcg/kg) | 200mcg over 15s (paediatrics: 10mcg/kg max. single dose 200mcg) |
| **Further IV doses as required** | 0.4–2mg every 2min (paediatrics: 100mcg/kg once, then question diagnosis) | 100–200mcg every 1min (paediatrics: 10mcg/kg repeated every 1min max. single dose 200mcg) |
| **Maximum total dose** | 10mg (consider alternative diagnosis if no response) | 1mg (consider alternative diagnosis if no response) |

**Patient comfort during procedure**

- An uncomfortable patient will require more sedation/analgesia.
- Careful patient positioning is essential, especially for long procedures.
  - Ensure patient is in a comfortable position before starting.
  - Arthritic pain from lying still can be more painful than the procedure itself.
  - Many patients are unable to lie flat for a prolonged time due to cardiorespiratory disease or severe reflux and need to be propped up slightly.
  - Consider lowering ischaemic feet into a dependent position for parts of procedures if pain is problematic.

- • Protect pressure areas.
- • Some patients tolerate the claustrophobia of MRI better if lying prone.
- Keep patients warm.
- Consider urinary catheterization for planned long procedures.

## Post sedation care

- Patients should be recovered by trained staff in a dedicated, suitably equipped recovery area within the department.
- If the patient is being transferred within the hospital before fully recovered (i.e. awake, orientated, haemodynamically stable and without respiratory compromise) they must be accompanied by a suitably trained member of staff and appropriate monitoring.
- Patients going home must be accompanied by a responsible adult overnight, have access to a telephone at home, be within a relatively short distance travelling from the hospital and have suitable travel arrangements.
- Any specific post procedure care requirements must be fully documented and explained to the patient/carer.
- Patients should avoid any activity which might be impaired by the residual effects of the drugs for at least 24hrs, e.g. driving, making important decisions.

## Additional paediatric considerations

- Experienced staff, appropriate patient selection and a quiet child-friendly environment are key features for success.
- A deeper level of sedation is generally necessary so that the child remains asleep for the entire procedure. They are not expected to be able to respond to verbal stimuli.
- No airway intervention should be required but those administering this type of sedation must be skilled in advanced paediatric airway management and life support.
- Many hospitals have paediatric sedation protocols and some have multidisciplinary sedation teams.
- General anaesthesia or anaesthetist-supervised sedation may be more appropriate for patients with contraindications or cautions to sedation and for procedures likely to be painful or to induce autonomic reflexes.
- Patients frequently have multiple scans. Old notes and parents can give valuable information as to the most suitable technique for that child.

**Contraindications to sedation in children[3]**
- Abnormal airway
- Raised intracranial pressure
- Depressed conscious level
- History of sleep apnoea
- Respiratory failure
- Cardiac failure
- Neuromuscular disease
- Bowel obstruction
- Acute respiratory tract infection
- Known allergy or adverse reaction to sedative
- Child too distressed despite adequate preparation
- Older children with severe behavioural problems
- Consent refusal by parent or patient

**Extra caution with**
- Neonates (especially if premature or ex-premature)
- Infants and children <5 years
- Children with impaired cardiac, renal or hepatic function
- Anticonvulsant therapy
- Respiratory disease
- Gastro-oesophageal reflux
- Impaired bulbar function
- Emergency cases
- Children already receiving opioids, other sedatives or drugs which potentiate the action of sedatives

- Infants under 4 months of age will tend to sleep through a scan if recently fed and wrapped up well.
- Fasting pre sedation: 6hrs for solids or formula milk, 4hrs for breast milk, 2hrs for clear fluid (oral contrast for bowel opacification for CT e.g. diluted Iohexol or Iopamidol is classed as clear fluid).

**Commonly used oral sedative drugs (paediatrics)**
- Midazolam
  - Benzodiazepine. No analgesic effect.
  - Amnesic and anxiolytic effect greater than sedative effect.
  - Sedative effects may be unpredictable. Can cause paradoxical agitation in higher doses.
  - Suitable for children >1 year of age undergoing brief procedures
  - Presentation: use IV solution for injection orally—1mg/ml, 2mg/ml or 5mg/ml (tastes bitter so mix with cordial/juice).
  - Dose PO: 0.5mg/kg (max 20mg).
  - Onset of effect: 30–60min.
  - Can be given buccally or intranasally (dose 0.2mg/kg). The nasal route stings and absorption is rapid leading to occasional apnoea and desaturation.

- Chloral hydrate or its active metabolite triclofos
  - Hypnotic
  - No analgesic effect
  - Used for many years in children <2 years of age
  - Main side-effect is gastric irritation and sometimes vomiting. Triclofos is better tolerated in this respect.
  - Presentation: Chloral hydrate: oral solution 143.3mg/5ml, 200mg/5ml or 500mg/5ml. Triclofos: 500mg/5ml
  - Dose PO: 30–50mg/kg (up to 100mg/kg (max 2mg) in some circumstances)
  - Onset of effect: 45–60min
  - Duration of action longer than midazolam
- Alternatives include temazepam and melatonin.


- Intravenous sedation should only be given by an anaesthetist.
- Sedation may fail in some patients due to patient variability and the need to maintain a margin of safety.


## Further reading

**1.** The Wylie Report: Report of the working party on Training in Dental Anaesthesia (1981) *Br Dental J* **151**; 385–8.

**2.** The Association of Anaesthetists of Great Britain & Ireland (2007) *Guidelines for the management of severe local anaesthetic toxicity*. London: AAGBI. Also available at http://www.aagbi.org/publications/guidelines/docs/latoxicity07.pdf (Accessed 24 June 2008).

**3.** SIGN (2002) *Safe sedation of children undergoing diagnostic and therapeutic procedures. A national guideline*. Scottish Intercollegiate Guidelines Network. http://www.sign.ac.uk/guidelines/fulltext/58/index.html.

**4.** Board of the Faculty of Clinical Radiology of the Royal College of Radiologists (2003) *Safe sedation, analgesia, and anaesthesia within the radiology department*. London: Royal College of Radiologists.

**5.** Intercollegiate working party chaired by the Royal College of Anaesthetists (2001) *Implementing and ensuring safe sedation practice for healthcare procedures in adults*. London: Royal College of Anaesthetists.

# Management of the paediatric patient

Acutely unwell children are usually frightened and in pain, which can make imaging difficult and traumatic for all involved. All radiology departments that image children should have rooms designed to be child friendly. Whenever possible you should use these facilities.

## General points

When imaging babies and young children explain to the parents what you are going to do and ask them to stay with their child. Children are very good at sensing their parents' anxieties. Calm parents who can reassure their child are your most valued asset. Paediatric rooms often have a selection of toys and a paediatric nurse or play specialist can also help by distracting the child. Lights on the ceiling, projectors and televisions are commonly used in ultrasound rooms and are very effective. In screening rooms, light projectors and music work best.

When dealing with older children try to explain in such a way that they can understand what you are going to do and how you want them to help. If you are going to do something that might be painful (such as removing a dressing) it is best to warn them first. If you do it without warning, or if try to be kind by telling them it won't hurt, you risk losing their trust and co-operation. In older children getting them to choose the music or video to be played can be helpful.

Children have a short attention span and small babies get cold very quickly so it is best to set the room up in advance of their arrival. If possible, raise the temperature to a level that will be comfortable for them for the amount of clothing covering them during the procedure.

## Ultrasound

When setting up the ultrasound room always put an absorbent pad on the bed as it will save the need for clearing spills after the procedure. Everyone has their own routine when performing an ultrasound scan but with children it is not always possible to adhere to this. Unfortunately this may make it more likely that you will forget part of the study, so check your images before the patient leaves. When scanning children, their small size allows the use of higher frequency probes which gives higher resolution images. Select the probe according to the patient's size to give a balance of image resolution and depth of penetration.

Children are often reluctant to lie down and it can help to start the ultrasound with the patient sitting on their parent's lap. If the abdomen is tender in one area, start with the other side to allow the child to become relaxed and then move to the painful area last. Leave the nappy on a baby whenever possible; it is usually only necessary to undo one side of the nappy to scan the bladder.

In some patients reassurance and distraction do not work, in which case it is often necessary to ask the parents or an accompanying nurse to hold the patient whilst you perform the study as best and as rapidly as is possible given the difficult circumstances.

It is important to store plenty of images, especially if you intend to discuss the ultrasound with a paediatric radiologist at a later time.

## Fluoroscopy

To reduce the radiation exposure, select a low-dose fluoroscopy setting with a low pulse rate. In babies and infants there is little scatter because of their small size and a grid is not usually needed. In most cases, all the required information can be obtained from stored fluoroscopic images without the need for formal radiographs (or exposures). Some departments record the entire screening case on video to allow later review. Local protocols should always be considered.

The radiology staff and the parents will need to wear lead coats: brightly coloured and patterned ones or those with pictures and cartoons are less intimidating than the lead coats normally used for adult fluoroscopy. Ask the parents to stand at the head of the table where the child can see them. Parents can help to hold and distract their child and can feed them the contrast medium during an upper gastrointestinal (GI) tract study.

If the procedure is going to involve moving the child, tell the parents exactly what you want them to do before you start. This is particularly important in the upper GI study when you want to turn the child supine quickly and accurately.

# Imaging strategies

Richard Graham
Ferdia Gallagher

Nyree Griffin

# Head and facial imaging

## Imaging modalities

### Radiographs

#### Skull radiographs (SXR)

Radiographs of the skull have no role in the diagnosis of significant brain injury. However, they are useful as part of the skeletal survey in children presenting with suspected non-accidental injury.

In some centres where CT access is limited, plain film is used to detect skull fractures but clearly any possible underlying brain injury cannot be evaluated and therefore plain skull radiographs are not advocated in normal practice.

#### Facial X-ray

When facial fractures are suspected the following recommended is:
- Occipitomental (OM) view.
- Occipitomental 30° (OM30) view.

### CT

#### Head CT

Unenhanced head CT is the mainstay for emergency head imaging. There are two basic protocols:
- Single slice acquisition with the tube angled along a line drawn from the external auditory meati (EAMs) to the superior orbital ridge (about 23°). Thin slices through the skull base and posterior fossa (e.g. 4mm) and thicker slices through the cranial vault (e.g. 10mm).
- Spiral acquisition with thin slice thickness (e.g. acquire at 5mm using 0.75mm detector and reconstruct into 1mm slices at 0.7mm interval) through the head without tube angulation.

Which protocol you choose will depend on the equipment in your institution and local practice. In general, spiral acquisition will be used for multidetector CT (MDCT) with 16 or more slices as it allows multiplanar reformats to be performed and this will increase the ease of detection of skull and facial fractures.

Although intravenous contrast is generally not needed in the emergency setting, it is useful in the following indications:
- To rule out cerebral metastases
- To further evaluate a space-occupying lesion detected on NECT
- To rule out venous sinus thrombosis
- For CT angiography of the cerebral circulation

Checklist for reviewing a head CT to avoid the commonly missed abnormalities. Such an approach is particularly important in the unconscious patient:

**Assessment for extra-axial collections, e.g. subdural or extradural haemorrhage:**
- Alter the window settings used to display the image—exclude a collection of similar intensity to the adjacent brain or CSF.
- Check the position of the brain cortex: is it displaced by a mass?
- Look either side of the falx.
- Look at the tentorium.
- Look in the middle cerebral fossa.
- Look at the inferior frontal region.
- Consider giving contrast medium.
- Consider reformatting the images (if thin slice acquisition has been used) and review sagittal and coronal images.

**Assessment for subarachnoid haemorrhage; common areas for blood:**
- Anterior interhemispheric fissure.
- Sylvian fissures: ensure that they can easily be seen.
- Lateral ventricles: blood will collect in the occipital horns when supine.
- Third and fourth ventricles.
- Between the cerebral peduncles.
- Cerebellopontine angles.
- At the foramen magnum.

**Assessment for brain oedema or swelling:**
- Is the brain cortex easily visible throughout?
- Are the basal ganglia visible?
- Are the sulci effaced (narrowed or compressed) or displaced?
- Is there uncal herniation?
- Are any of the ventricles deformed or displaced?

**Assessment for dural venous sinus thrombosis:**
- How dense are the sinuses?
- Particularly assess the straight sinus.
- Have a low threshold for giving contrast medium or performing CT venography.

**Assessment of the ventricles:**
- Are they deformed or displaced?
- Do they contain blood or debris, particularly occipital horns?
- Is there transependymal oedema?
- Is there ependymal enhancement following contrast medium?

**Assessment of bones and soft tissues:**
- View images on bone window settings to assess for fractures and metastases.
- View images at soft tissue settings to assess for swelling which may help to identify the site of an underlying bone abnormality.
- The orbits should always be reviewed.

Adapted from reference 4.

### Facial CT

Spiral acquisition from the hard palate to the superior border of the orbits. No gantry angulation. 3mm slices using thinnest detector (e.g. 0.75mm). Reconstruct at 1mm slices with 0.7mm gap on soft tissue and bone algorithms. View with multiplanar reformatted images (MPR).

### MRI

Head (and cervical spine) MRI is contraindicated unless there is absolute certainty that the patient does not have an incompatible device, implant or foreign body.

# Indications for emergency head CT

The indications for head imaging are best considered as either traumatic or atraumatic. The latter category can be usefully subdivided into vascular and non-vascular problems. Following this, two common specific indications for head CT will be considered which frequently pose challenges for clinicians and radiologists: acute confusion and fitting/epilepsy.

## Traumatic

Head CT is the mainstay for imaging in the setting of trauma. A head CT should be extended to include the face if the clinician is concerned about facial fractures. Often it is appropriate to image the cervical spine at the same time (📖 p. 54). The NICE head injury guidelines[1] are listed in figure 4.1 and these are increasingly being implemented in the UK.

**In general, we need to image most patients who have suspected head trauma within 1hr. However, there is a small subset of patients who are <65 years old and present with normal neurological signs in whom imaging may be delayed by up to 8hrs from the time of injury. Additionally, if patients present out of hours and is ≥ 65, has amnesia for events more than 30 minutes before impact or there was a dangerous mechanism of injury, it is acceptable to admit for overnight observation, with CT imaging the next morning unless CT results are required within 1 hour because of the presence of additional clinical findings listed in figure 4.1**

Clearly each case must be considered in light of the individual patient's history and after discussion with the clinician managing the patient: for instance it may be inappropriate to CT a patient who is undergoing palliative care for metastatic disease even if they do fulfill the other criteria for imaging.

## NICE indications for CT imaging of the head following trauma

(a)

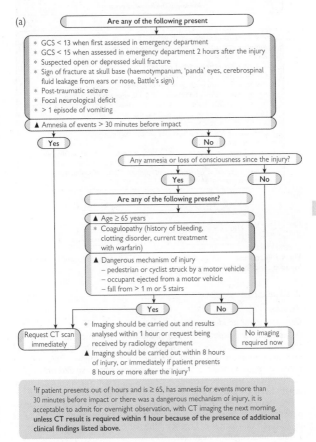

**Are any of the following present**

* GCS < 13 when first assessed in emergency department
* GCS < 15 when assessed in emergency department 2 hours after the injury
* Suspected open or depressed skull fracture
* Sign of fracture at skull base (haemotympanum, 'panda' eyes, cerebrospinal fluid leakage from ears or nose, Battle's sign)
* Post-traumatic seizure
* Focal neurological deficit
* > 1 episode of vomiting
▲ Amnesia of events > 30 minutes before impact

Yes — No

Any amnesia or loss of consciousness since the injury?

Yes — No

**Are any of the following present?**

▲ Age ≥ 65 years
* Coagulopathy (history of bleeding, clotting disorder, current treatment with warfarin)
▲ Dangerous mechanism of injury
  – pedestrian or cyclist struck by a motor vehicle
  – occupant ejected from a motor vehicle
  – fall from > 1 m or 5 stairs

Yes — No

Request CT scan immediately

* Imaging should be carried out and results analysed within 1 hour or request being received by radiology department
▲ Imaging should be carried out within 8 hours of injury, or immediately if patient presents 8 hours or more after the injury[1]

No imaging required now

[1]If patient presents out of hours and is ≥ 65, has amnesia for events more than 30 minutes before impact or there was a dangerous mechanism of injury, it is acceptable to admit for overnight observation, with CT imaging the next morning, **unless CT result is required within 1 hour because of the presence of additional clinical findings listed above.**

**Fig. 4.1** NICE guidelines for cranial CT imaging following trauma in (a) adults and (b) children.

(b)

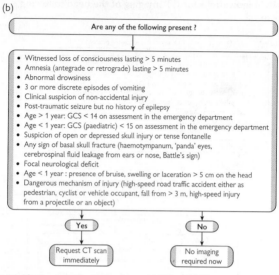

Are any of the following present ?

- Witnessed loss of consciousness lasting > 5 minutes
- Amnesia (antegrade or retrograde) lasting > 5 minutes
- Abnormal drowsiness
- 3 or more discrete episodes of vomiting
- Clinical suspicion of non-accidental injury
- Post-traumatic seizure but no history of epilepsy
- Age > 1 year: GCS < 14 on assessment in the emergency department
- Age < 1 year: GCS (paediatric) < 15 on assessment in the emergency department
- Suspicion of open or depressed skull injury or tense fontanelle
- Any sign of basal skull fracture (haemotympanum, 'panda' eyes, cerebrospinal fluid leakage from ears or nose, Battle's sign)
- Focal neurological deficit
- Age < 1 year : presence of bruise, swelling or laceration > 5 cm on the head
- Dangerous mechanism of injury (high-speed road traffic accident either as pedestrian, cyclist or vehicle occupant, fall from > 3 m, high-speed injury from a projectile or an object)

Yes → Request CT scan immediately

No → No imaging required now

**Fig. 4.1** (*Continued*) NICE guidelines for cranial CT imaging following trauma in (a) adults and (b) children.

## Atraumatic

### Vascular[2,3]

#### Cerebrovascular accident

Assessment for suspected stroke is the main indication for head CT in the atraumatic category. The reason to image stroke acutely is to differentiate haemorrhagic from non-haemorrhagic stroke. This differentiation is required prior to treating non-haemorrhagic stroke with aspirin. Furthermore, as stroke thrombolysis services are increasingly established, urgent head CT imaging will be needed to identify suitable candidates.

Brain imaging should be undertaken as soon as possible in all stroke patients and at least within 24hrs of onset of symptoms. It should be undertaken as a matter of urgency if the patient has:

- Taken anticoagulant treatment
- A known bleeding tendency
- A depressed level of consciousness
- Unexplained progressive or fluctuating symptoms
- Papilloedema, neck stiffness or fever
- Severe headache at onset
- Indications for early anticoagulation

#### Indications for thrombolysis

- Acute ischaemic stroke within 3hrs of symptom onset and with a clinically meaningful neurologic deficit

- Baseline brain CT or other diagnostic imaging method (MRI) showing no evidence of intracranial hemorrhage

*Contraindications for thrombolysis include*
- Intracranial haemorrhage
- Involvement of more than 1/3 of the MCA territory on the initial CT
- Seizure at stroke onset
- Prior stroke in the last 3 months
- Heparin treatment in last 48hrs and activated partial thromboplastin time above upper limit of normal
- Thrombocytopaenia (platelets <100 000/mm$^3$)
- Systolic BP >185 mmHg or diastolic >110 mmHg
- Blood glucose <2.8mmol/L or >22mmol/L

If the underlying pathology is uncertain, or the diagnosis of stroke is in doubt after CT head, MRI should be considered (this can generally wait until normal working hours).

### Venous sinus and cerebral vein thrombosis

The clinical presentation is non-specific but often includes headache, vomiting and papilloedema. Depending on which sinus is involved (often several are involved), the signs and symptoms differ (📖 p. 212). If the clinician suspects it, then the radiologist needs to carefully consider it on review of the imaging. Magnetic resonance venogram (MRV) is the imaging investigation of choice but is often unavailable in the emergency setting when a cranial CT before and after IV contrast medium is generally used.

### Cerebral haemorrhage

*Subarachnoid haemorrhage*

Subarachnoid haemorrhage (SAH) should be considered in any patient presenting with a sudden onset of severe and unusual headache, with or without any associated alteration in consciousness. CT does not exclude subarachnoid haemorrhage as 2% of SAH are CT negative and a lumbar puncture must be performed if the CT demonstrates no haemorrhage.

It is usual for computed tomography angiography (CTA) and/or magnetic resonance angiography (MRA) to be performed subsequently to elucidate the aetiology of the haemorrhage.

*Extradural haemorrhage*

95% are associated with skull fractures. Large extradural haemorrhages are a neurosurgical emergency. CT should be performed immediately if suspected.

*Subdural haemorrhage*

Not generally associated with skull fractures. Common in non-accidental injury (NAI) and the elderly. The symptoms on presentation are often like those of a space-occupying lesion (SOL). CT should be performed if suspected.

### Non-vascular

### Meningitis and encephalitis

The reason to perform a CT head in meningitis is to exclude signs of raised intracranial pressure prior to lumbar puncture. Although head CT is not a surrogate measure of intracranial pressure, there are imaging features that would make one concerned about the patient undergoing lumbar puncture (LP) (📖 p. 232 in neuro meningitis section). In encephalitis, head CT is often normal but there may be asymmetric areas of low attenuation in the temporal lobes with loss of grey/white matter differentiation. MRI is the investigation of choice but is generally not available in the emergency setting.

### Space-occupying lesion

Head CT is a good way to diagnose SOL in the acute situation. IV contrast medium is usually given to characterize the lesion further. Patients who have SOLs will often have an MRI subsequently for further characterization of the lesion.

## Acute confusion

The main organic diagnoses that should be excluded with CT are:
• Space occupying lesion
• Stroke
• Hydrocephalus
• Subdural haemorrhage (SDH)

## Epilepsy

NICE has provided guildelines on imaging following a fit/epilepsy.[5] CT and MRI are used to identify structural abnormalities that cause certain epilepsies. Acute imaging is not generally indicated when the patient has a known diagnosis of idiopathic generalized epilepsy.

In the acute setting CT can be indicated to determine whether a seizure has been caused by an acute neurological lesion or illness. CT is also indicated for definitive imaging (in the non-emergency setting) if MRI is contraindicated or unavailable.

MRI is the imaging investigation of choice for people with epilepsy. The use of MRI is particularly important for people:
• Who have developed epilepsy as adults
• Who have any suggestion of a focal onset from history, examination or EEG
• In whom seizures continue in spite of first-line medication

MRI should be performed within 4 weeks of request rather than as an emergency.

# Indications for facial imaging

## Plain film

Plain films are indicated when facial fractures are suspected. Plain films are not indicated for suspected nasal fractures.

## CT

Facial CT has two main indications in emergency radiology:
- To characterize complex facial fractures for pre-operation planning
- To rule out retrobulbar involvement in peri-orbital cellulitis

## Further reading

**1.** NICE (2007) *Head Injury Guidelines*, available at http://www.nice.org.uk/guidance/index.jsp?action=download&o=36259.

**2.** RCP ( 2004) Intercollegiate Stroke Working Party (2004) *RCP National Clinical Guidelines for Stroke*, 2nd edn, available at http://www.rcplondon.ac.uk/pubs/books/stroke/.

**3.** Thrombolysis Interest Group of Canada Guidelines, April 2007 http://www.tigc.org/eguidelines/thrombolysisacutestroke07.htm

**4.** Harden SP, Dey C, Gawne-Cain Ml (2007) Cranial CT of the unconscious patient. *Clinical Radiology* **62**; 404–15.

**5.** NICE (2004) *The Epilepsies: Diagnosis and Management of the Epilepsies in Adults in Primary and Secondary Care*, available at http://www.nice.org.uk/guidance/index.jsp?action=byID&r-true&o10954.

# Spinal imaging

## Imaging modalities

### Cervical spine

*Radiographs*

The current initial investigation of choice for the detection of injuries to the cervical spine is the three-view radiograph series:
- Lateral
- Anteroposterior (AP)
- Open-mouth peg view

These must be of good technical quality:
- AP and lateral should show C7/T1 junction
- Peg view should show C1 and C2 clearly

### CT

Thin slices (e.g. acquire at 3mm, reconstruct at 1mm thickness with 0.7mm gap) are acquired in a spiral acquisition. The extent of the imaging should be from base of skull to the lower border of T1 vertebral body in the patient with a GCS = 15 and to the lower border of T4 if the GCS is <15. This is because the T1–T4 vertebrae are very difficult to assess using plain film. If CT is being performed for inadequate or abnormal plain films it is advisable to image the entire C-spine rather than just the level of interest as this allows a complete and accurate assessment of the whole C-spine to be made.

> **Checklist for reviewing a C-spine CT to avoid the commonly missed abnormalities**
> - Assess the adequacy of the images i.e. has C1–T1 (or even lower if appropriate) been imaged.
> - Review multiplanar reformatted images on bone window settings.
> - Compare any suspected abnormality with the opposite side for symmetry.
> - Always look beyond the spine: soft tissue swelling may help to identify a fracture. Assess for features of ligamentous injury without a fracture, e.g. malalignment of the vertebral bodies or spinous processes.
> - Review the lung apices (if imaged) on lung window settings.
> - Review the sternum and ribs
> - Review the scout image for fractures outside the axial CT field of view e.g. glenoid fracture

### Thoracic spine

*X-ray*

Plain films (AP and lateral views) are the mainstay for thoracic spine imaging in trauma. It is difficult to clear from T1 to T4 due to superimposition of the shoulders; although swimmer's views and oblique views can be used, CT is the best modality for imaging the upper thoracic spine.

*CT*

When a thoracic spine abnormality is suspected, it is usually necessary to exclude other thoracic abnormalities with a chest CT (📖 p. 58). Therefore the thoracic spine is usually assessed with a bony reconstruction of the chest CT data thus obviating the need for further imaging of the thoracic spine.

It is vital to view reformats of the thoracic CT in the three anatomical planes to increase diagnostic certainty.

### Lumbar spine and sacrum
*X-ray*

AP and lateral views are usually acquired.

*CT*

If CT of the abdomen and pelvis (📖 p. 68) is being performed, a bony reconstruction of the lumbar spine and sacrum can be obtained from this data set without the need for further specific imaging of the lumbar spine.

*MRI*

Usually only acquired in the emergency setting to evaluate spinal cord compression or cauda equina syndrome.

A suggested protocol includes sagittal $T_1$ and $T_2$ or $T_1$ and short tau inversion recovery (STIR) imaging. Axial $T_2$ and $T_1$ images through any abnormal area can be subsequently acquired. The choice of sequences will usually depend on local experience and hardware performance.

# Indications for spinal imaging

## Trauma

### Cervical spine

Generally CT is used if the plain films are:

- Inadequate
- Normal but there is still high clinical suspicion
- Impossible to obtain because the patient's GCS is too low
- Definitive imaging is needed urgently (e.g. 8hr surgical procedure about to commence on another part of the body)

## NICE guidelines for cervical spine imaging in trauma

The NICE head injury guidelines are followed in the UK and list indications for C-spine imaging in trauma. They are reproduced below.

Children aged 10 years or more can be treated as adults for the purposes of C-spine imaging.

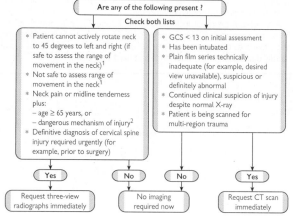

**Fig. 4.2** Criteria for C-spine imaging for adults and children aged 10 years or more.

**1.** Safe assessment can be carried out if patient: was involved in a simple rear-end motor vehical collision; is comfortable in a sitting position in the emergency department; has been ambulatory at any time since injury and there is no midline cervical spine tenderness; or if the patient presents with delayed onset of neck pain.

**2.** Dangerous mechanism of injury: fall from > 1 m or 5 stairs; axial load to head – for example, diving; high-speed motor vehicle collision; rollover motor accident; ejection from a motor vehicle; accident involving motorized recreational vehicles: bicycle collision.

Children under 10 years should receive AP and lateral views without an AP peg view. Abnormalities or uncertainties in those under 10 years should be clarified by CT imaging. When minor trauma is associated with subsequent torticollis the plain films are almost uninterpretable; CT is very helpful in this situation.

In children under 10 years, CT of the cervical spine should be used with caution because of the increased risks associated with irradiation (particularly to the thyroid gland) and the lower risk of significant spinal injury in general. Indications include:

- Severe head injury (GCS ≤8)
- A strong suspicion of injury despite normal plain films, or cases where there is a strong suspicion of injury and plain films are inadequate.
- CT should also be undertaken when the GCS is between 9 and 14 if there is high clinical concern (for example, focal neurological deficit or paraesthesia in the extremities).

### Timing

- Imaging of the cervical spine should be performed within 1hr of a request having been received by the radiology department.
- Where a request for urgent head CT (i.e. within 1hr) has also been received, the C-spine imaging should also be carried out within 1hr.
- Children less than 10 years old who have a GCS of 8 or less should have a CT of the C-spine within 1hr of presentation.

### Thoracic spine

The indications for CT are:

- If there is a suspected T1–T4 fracture, in patients who have a GCS <15. The thoracic spine CT should be performed in conjunction with the C-spine CT.
- To evaluate an abnormality identified on plain film: it is usual to image the area of concern with CT.
- Inability to obtain adequate plain films.

### Lumbar spine and sacrum

Plain film is indicated in the evaluation of trauma to the lumbar spine and sacrum. The indications for CT are:

- Inability to obtain adequate plain films
- To evaluate abnormalities detected on plain film

## Atraumatic

### Spinal cord and cauda equina compression

Usually presents with leg weakness. There may also be urinary retention and faecal incontinence. It is important to image early to avoid irreversible neural damage. MRI is the imaging modality of choice as the diagnosis cannot be excluded on CT.

# Thoracic imaging

## Imaging modalities

### Radiographs

#### Chest radiographs (CXR)

This is the primary imaging investigation for most suspected thoracic abnormalities. However, imaging should not delay emergency treatment: for example in cases where tension pneumothorax is suspected, emergency decompression of the pleural space should precede any imaging.

- Where possible, a posteroanterior (PA) film should be obtained in the radiology department.
- Frequently in the emergency setting a portable supine AP film is all that can be obtained; this may be of poor quality due to movement artefact, inadequate positioning, rotation of the patient and inadequate exposure due to the suboptimal conditions for image acquisiton. Despite this, the CXR is still recommended as a first line investigation in most trauma management guidelines.[1,2] Both the emergency physician and the radiologist must be aware of the inherent limitations of these portable films: for instance the sensitivity of detecting a pneumothorax on supine CXR can be as low as 50% (📖 p. 90) and further imaging, such as an erect departmental PA CXR or CT,[1] should always be considered.
- An expiratory CXR can be used to increase the sensitivity of detecting air trapping, particularly following suspected inhalation of a foreign body. It may also enhance the demonstration of a small pneumothorax.[3]
- While the lateral CXR has a role in elective thoracic imaging, it is increasingly common for abnormalities of uncertain significance on frontal CXR to be evaluated with CT in the emergency setting. However, a lateral film is often used to exclude a fracture of the sternum.[1]

### Ultrasound

The major role for ultrasound (US) is in the evaluation of pleural collections or effusions as well as for guided aspiration and drainage (📖 p. 374). US may also be useful to evaluate the nature of a soft tissue collection such as a breast abscess (📖 p. 332). Doppler US of the axillary and subclavian veins can be used to assess for deep vein thrombosis of the upper limb but the overlying clavicles can limit visualization of the subclavian vein.

- 4–6 MHz curvilinear probes are usually used for chest ultrasound, ideally with the patient in the sitting position for assessment of a pleural collection.
- 8–10 MHz linear probe for Doppler vascular imaging.

### CT

High resolution MDCT can now produce isotropic voxels (i.e. the voxel has the same dimensions in all three directions). The resulting data can be viewed in the three main anatomical planes with the same spatial resolution (often 1mm or less). This post-processing technique is known as multiplanar reformatting, also the data can be manipulated to enhance the appearance of vessels–maximum intensity projections (MIPs) (see Fig. 4.3). Multiplanar reformatted images (MPRs) greatly assist in the diagnosis of thoracic and abdominal abnormalities and allow data sets to be viewed in an anatomically intuitive way: surgeons are accustomed to viewing the body in the coronal plane during surgery and imaging presented in this format is usually easier for them to appreciate than traditional axial images.

CT has become increasingly central to the management of emergency patients who are stable and have immediately non life-threatening problems. The following is an outline of the common CT protocols used in emergency thoracic imaging; in all cases there will be regional variation and local departmental guidelines should be followed.

### Non-enhanced CT (NECT)

- The thorax is imaged if possible in a single breath hold and normally in a caudal to cranial direction. Contiguous images are acquired.
- The images should include the entire lungs: from the apices to costophrenic angles. The radiographer should ensure that this is the case before the patient is removed from the CT table.
- With current MDCT technology, slices are usually reconstructed at 2.5–5mm. Thinner reconstructions can be used to evaluate fine morphological detail, e.g. the lung parenchyma.
- The role of the thoracic NECT is limited in the emergency setting but should be considered for the assessment of haemorrhage prior to the administration of contrast medium, e.g. following trauma or when the patient is being evaluated for aortic dissection. However, in children and pregnant women the small potential benefit of such a study must be balanced against the increased radiation exposure, and in these cases a contrast enhanced study acquired in a single phase may be sufficient.

### Contrast enhanced CT (CECT)

- Images are acquired in a similar manner to the NECT but following IV iodinated contrast medium, e.g. 70–100ml at 2–5ml/s for adults. The patient will therefore require an IV cannula and ideally this should be sited prior to arrival in the radiology department. The right antecubital fossa is the best location as this will avoid the potential streak artefact from opacification of the left brachicocephalic vein as it traverses the superior mediastinum. Renal function should be noted prior to administration and any history of previous allergy to contrast medium should be elicited. If the patient has impaired renal function, then a discussion with the referring team is essential: please see Chapter 2 for further considerations before giving contrast medium.
- Images are usually acquired either in a pulmonary arterial phase (see CTPA below) or in a systemic arterial phase.
- There are several methods for determining the time from the start of contrast medium injection to image acquisition:
  - The study can be *bolus triggered* as the contrast medium enters the vessel in question: ascending aorta or pulmonary trunk. A region of interest is placed over the vessel which is continuously imaging until the density of contrast within it reaches a predefined threshold.

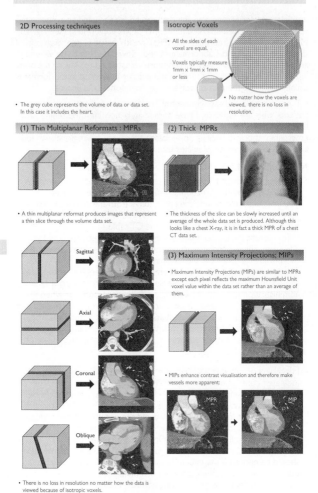

**2D Processing techniques**

- The grey cube represents the volume of data or data set. In this case it includes the heart.

**Isotropic Voxels**

- All the sides of each voxel are equal.

  Voxels typically measure 1mm x 1mm x 1mm or less

- No matter how the voxels are viewed, there is no loss in resolution.

**(1) Thin Multiplanar Reformats : MPRs**

- A thin multiplanar reformat produces images that represent a thin slice through the volume data set.

**(2) Thick MPRs**

- The thickness of the slice can be slowly increased until an average of the whole data set is produced. Although this looks like a chest X-ray, it is in fact a thick MPR of a chest CT data set.

**(3) Maximum Intensity Projections; MIPs**

- Maximum Intensity Projections (MIPs) are similar to MPRs except each pixel reflects the maximum Hounsfield Unit voxel value within the data set rather than an average of them.

- MIPs enhance contrast visualisation and therefore make vessels more apparent.

Sagittal

Axial

Coronal

Oblique

- There is no loss in resolution no matter how the data is viewed because of isotropic voxels.

**Fig. 4.3** Two-dimensional post-processing techniques. Schematic showing how isotropic voxels from a CT dataset can be used to create (1) Thin MPRs; (2) Thick MPRs; and (3) MIPs.

- A variation of this involves a *test bolus* where the time taken for a small volume (20ml) of contrast medium to reach the vessel of interest is measured. This figure is used to determine the length of time between the full dose of contrast medium and the image acquisition.
- Alternatively it can be triggered at a *fixed delay time* following injection: typically this is about 25–30s but delayed scanning at 40–50s may be useful in assessment of an empyema.
- Oral contrast medium is generally not given.
- A general protocol for an adult thoracic CT is 100mls of IV contrast medium (150mg iodine/ml) injected at a rate of 2.5ml/s after a 25s delay.[3]

## CT pulmonary angiogram (CTPA)

This is used in the evaluation of pulmonary emboli to produce an image of the pulmonary arterial tree

- To accurately diagnose or exclude a pulmonary embolism, the HU density of the pulmonary artery should be >230; between 200–230 it is regarded as suboptimal; and below <200 it is non-diagnostic.
- A typical protocol involves a uniphasic bolus injection of 370mg iodine/ml at 4ml/s with a 20s delay. If possible, imaging is performed within a single breath hold.
- Alternatively, bolus tracking may be used with the region of interest set over the pulmonary trunk.

## High resolution CT (HRCT)

HRCT images are used to demonstrate the lung parenchyma. They were traditionally acquired as non-contiguous 1–2mm slices 20–30mm apart. The high spatial resolution that is now possible with current MDCTs allows the entire chest to be reconstructed into contiguous 1mm slices and therefore HRCT is often no longer performed as a separate investigation. Furthermore, although traditionally no contrast medium was used, current MDCT practice is usually to acquire a single study post IV contrast medium: in addition to the volumetric chest data, 1mm slices can be reconstructed at 10mm intervals producing images that can used to assess the lung parenchyma. In conventional HRCT the whole chest is not imaged and the dose is therefore low: consequently small lung nodules may be missed if they lie between the imaged slices. Newer MDCT thoracic protocols image the whole chest so will not miss such nodules, but the dose is higher than with an HRCT.

The role of HRCT imaging in the emergency setting is limited but may be useful to help assess the cause of pulmonary consolidation.

## Cardiac CT and the future of acute chest pain imaging

Cardiac CT is a dedicated ECG-gated study to assess the heart and coronary vessels. Although currently not a routine emergency imaging tool, its use is increasing and it may replace assessment with coronary angiography in selected patient groups. The protocol includes:

- The field of view centred on the heart.
- ECG-gating.

- The initial low dose NECT gives a quantitative value for coronary calcium known as the *calcium score* which correlates with atherosclerotic plaque burden and gives prognostic information regarding future cardiovascular events.
- The subsequent CECT can be performed in a number of ways to evaluate the patency of the coronary arteries:
  - Give a test bolus of 20ml at 4ml/s.
  - Alternatively, bolus trigger the contrast medium at the aortic root.
  - Monophasic (140ml at 3ml/s) or biphasic injection (50ml at 4ml/s followed by 100ml at 2.5ml/s) can be used.
  - A saline flush or *chaser* is frequently used (40ml at 2.5ml/s).
- A low heart rate is ideal (<60 BPM) and short acting β-blockers are generally used to achieve this.
- Images are reconstructed at multiple points in the cardiac cycle.
- A normal CT coronary angiogram has a high negative predictive value (NPV) for exclusion of coronary artery disease in certain patient groups and may be used in the future to evaluate such patients' chest pain.

Advances in MDCT technology (particularly 64-slice MDCT and above) have made it possible for the entire chest to be imaged with ECG-gating in a single breath hold. This can allow simultaneous assessment of three major causes of chest pain: ischaemic heart disease, dissection and pulmonary embolus. In the future, such a protocol may become the first line imaging regime in patients with chest pain.

### Nuclear medicine

A ventilation (V)–perfusion (Q) study is used to assess pulmonary blood flow and alveolar ventilation. It is used as an alternative to CTPA to image pulmonary emboli (🕮 p. 85).
- Perfusion imaging is normally performed with $^{99m}$Technetium-labelled nanoparticles.
- Ventilation imaging can be performed with several gases such as $^{81m}$Krypton or $^{133}$Xenon.
- The diagnosis of a PE is based on perfusion defects that are not matched on ventilation.
- A half dose Q scan (with no ventilation imaging) may be used during pregnancy in order to reduce radiation burden (🕮 p. 87).

### Intervention

Arterial phase CT has largely superseded diagnostic arterial angiography for suspected aneurysmal or traumatic vascular leak of the thoracic aorta and other vessels. However, the emergency deployment of a covered stent may be used when the diagnosis has been made to avoid invasive surgery.

Similarly, CTPA has replaced the need for pulmonary angiography although the latter may still be used to demonstrate arteriovenous pulmonary malformations. Bronchial artery embolization is still occasionally used for life-threatening haemoptysis.

Coronary angiography plays a major role in acute chest management but is rarely performed by radiologists and will not be covered in this text (see companion volume *Emergencies in Cardiology*, OUP).

The use of image-guided aspiration or drainage of pleural collections with CT or US is increasing. Such procedures can be performed either on the ward with a hand-held miniature US (e.g. Sonosite®), with a portable high-resolution US, or alternatively in the radiology department.

## Other

- A water-soluble contrast swallow study may be used to assess for oesophageal perforation (📖 p. 180), fistula or post-operative leak.
- Gastrografin® should not be used due to the risk of aspiration.
- Patient should be examined semi-supine (20°).
- Imaging is performed in the left and right lateral positions.

MRI and PET of the thorax are not routinely used for emergency imaging.

> ### Checklist for reviewing a thoracic CT to avoid the commonly missed abnormalities
>
> - Assess the adequacy of the images, e.g. is the opacification of the pulmonary arteries sufficient to exclude a pulmonary embolism (PE) (see text for details).
> - Review images on lung, mediastinal and bone window settings (see Table 4.1).
> - Review multiplanar reformatted images particularly when assessing the spine for abnormalities.
> - Consider MIP imaging for the assessment of the pulmonary vasculature and for nodule detection.
> - Assess the large airways for narrowing, irregularity or the presence of a mass.
> - Carefully review each lung using the thin reconstructed axial images to exclude small pulmonary nodules.
> - Assess soft tissues, e.g. breasts, axillae and cervical region.
> - Pay particular attention to the heart even if cardiac gating has not been performed, as many abnormalities may still be detectable, e.g. pericardial effusions, left ventricular thinning or coronary calcification.
> - Review the limited images below the diaphragm e.g. for an adrenal mass.

# Indications for emergency thoracic CT

The indications for thoracic imaging have been divided into traumatic and atraumatic, with the latter further subdivided into vascular and non-vascular presentations.

## Traumatic

While a CXR is usually performed in patients presenting with thoracic trauma, the need for a subsequent thoracic CT should be considered in such patients. Although each case should be reviewed on an individual basis in accordance with local protocols, some general guidance is given below:

- Minor trauma: CT is rarely required.
- Moderate trauma in the stable patient: an erect PA CXR is needed to exclude a pneumothorax as well as to demonstrate pleural fluid or lung contusion. CT is useful for suspected aortic trauma and to exclude a pneumothorax not shown on a supine CXR.[1]
- Severe trauma: there should be a low threshold for urgent CT imaging of such patients, particularly those who have experienced rapid deceleration or penetrating injuries.
- Unstable patients: the patient should be stabilized before being transferred for imaging although portable imaging may be possible while the patient is being stabilized. Importantly, imaging should not delay life-saving treatment such as surgery.
- Simple rib fractures: alone they do not alter management but complications may need to be excluded (e.g. on CXR). Multiple fractures, e.g. a flail segment, may require CT assessment to assess for associated injuries.
- Stab injuries: a pneumothorax needs to be excluded. Depending on the depth and site of penetration, CT or US may be required to assess for pleural or pericardial fluid as well as for vascular damage.
- Sternal injuries: frontal and lateral CXR are required. Spinal and aortic injuries should be considered.[1]
- A mechanism of injury severe enough to require chest CT may also require an abdominal CT. Possible imaging of the head and cervical spine should also be considered. These should be discussed with the referring clinician before contrast medium has been administered as a single injection can be used to image the thorax, abdomen (and head).

An NECT is frequently performed as part of the thoracic trauma series, although this is controversial as many argue that most diagnoses can be made on a single-phase CECT without the need for further radiation exposure. If performed, an NECT can be used to identify intrathoracic haemorrhage which is of high attenuation.

An arterial phase CECT will identify vascular damage such as active bleeding, or a traumatic pseudoaneurysm. Delayed CT may be helpful if venous haemorrhage is suspected but is rarely used in practice.

## Atraumatic

### Vascular

*Thoracic aortic dissection and aneurysm rupture*
Both are radiological emergencies and urgent CT is required if suspected.

*Pulmonary embolus (PE)*
This usually presents to the radiology department as a clearly defined clinical question in a patient with a good history and known risk factors. The main imaging approaches involve either a CTPA or V/Q: local departmental guidelines as well British Thoracic Society guidelines should be considered and a discussion of this subject is found on 📖 p. 84. If a CTPA is performed and no PE is identified it is important to exclude other causes of chest pain:
- Aortic dissection
- Pneumothorax
- Pneumonia
- Pericardial effusion
- Coronary artery disease (if image quality will allow this)
- Bone fractures or metastases

### Non-vascular

For most non-vascular abnormalities, a NECT or HRCT of the thorax will be sufficient.

**Table 4.1** Examples of CT display settings used to optimize anatomical contrast for different body areas. Most manufacturers will suggest appropriate window settings for viewing the images

|  | Window level (HU) | Window width (HU) |
|---|---|---|
| Lung | −600 | 1200–1500 |
| Mediastinum | 20–40 | 300–500 |
| PE-specific | 100 | 700 |
| General abdomen | 20–35 | 400–500 |
| Liver | 40–60 | 160–250 |
| Cerebrum | 35–40 | 80–100 |
| Posterior fossa | 40 | 120 |
| Vertebrae/bone | 400–500 | 1500–2000 |

## Further reading

**1.** RCR (2007) *Making the best use of clinical radiology services: referral guidelines.* Royal College of Radiologists, London.

**2.** American College of Surgeons (2004) *Advanced Trauma Life Support (ATLS)*, 7th edition. Available at http://www.facs.org/trauma/atls/index.html.

**3.** *Grainger and Allison's Diagnostic Radiology: A Textbook of Medical Imaging*; 5th edn; 2007. Churchill Livingstone, Edinburgh.

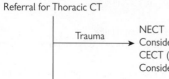

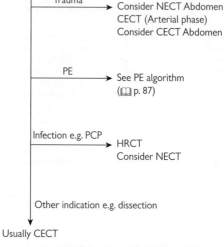

Referral for Thoracic CT

Trauma → NECT
Consider NECT Abdomen
CECT (Arterial phase)
Consider CECT Abdomen

PE → See PE algorithm
(📖 p. 87)

Infection e.g. PCP → HRCT
Consider NECT

Other indication e.g. dissection

Usually CECT

**Fig. 4.4** Suggested protocols for thoracic CT imaging depending on clinical presentation.

# Abdominal imaging

## Imaging modalities

### Radiographs

#### Abdominal radiographs (AXRs)

Although the AXR has traditionally been the primary imaging modality in patients presenting with abdominal pain, its role is diminishing as other modalities are increasing in importance.[1] Features to look for on AXR in the setting of the acute abdomen include:

- Free intra-abdominal air.
- Bowel dilatation due to:
  - mechanical obstruction
  - paralytic ileus
  - air swallowing
- Abdominal calcification, e.g.:
  - gallstones
  - renal tract calcification
  - appendicolith
  - calcified aneurysm
  - pancreatic calcification associated with pancreatitis
- Intramural gas, e.g.:
  - emphysematous cholecystitis
  - emphysematous gastritis
- Abdominal masses e.g. abdominal aortic aneurysm

### US

Abdominal and pelvic ultrasound is usually performed using a 3–6 MHz curvilinear probe. Localized imaging, e.g of the right iliac fossa in cases of appendicitis, can be performed using a linear probe (6–15 MHz). Transvaginal US (TVUS) is a useful tool for the assessment of the pelvis.

The major advantage of US over other techniques is the lack of exposure to radiation, allowing it to be used when other modalities are relatively contraindicated, e.g. pregnancy and childhood. However, it is user-dependent and as images are acquired in real time, they are difficult to review retrospectively. As well as being excellent for assessing the intra-abdominal solid organs (i.e. liver, spleen, kidney), US can be used to diagnose or assess for:

- Renal obstruction and calculi
- Biliary tree abnormalities, e.g. cholecystitis, common bile duct (CBD) obstruction
- Vascular abnormalities, e.g. abdominal aortic aneurysm measurements, assessment of portal venous flow, hepatic arterial flow in a transplant patient
- Detection of fluid
- Pelvic abnormalities, e.g. ectopic pregnancy or ovarian pathology
- Can be used by an experienced radiologist for the detection of bowel abnormalities, e.g appendicitis or intussusception
- Guidance of interventional procedures, e.g. targeted biopsies or drain insertion
- Scrotal assessment

- Abdominal wall hernias
- Abdominal wall haemorrhage, e.g. rectus sheath haematoma

### Focused assessment with sonography for trauma (FAST)

FAST has almost replaced diagnostic peritoneal lavage as a means of rapidly assessing polytrauma patients in the emergency department. Its main purpose is in the detection of peritoneal fluid in trauma. It is performed by non-radiologically trained staff to allow rapid assessment of patients in the emergency department. It is important that clinicians performing such tests are aware of their limitations and should contact a radiologist if they detect an abnormality they are unfamiliar with. Patients with a positive FAST scan should be taken straight for exploratory laparotomy, or more fully assessed with CT, depending upon the clinical condition of the patient.

### CT

As with thoracic CT, abdominal CT has become increasingly central to the management of emergency abdominal problems. Once again, high-resolution MDCT has allowed images to be reviewed in all three anatomical planes. The following is an outline of the common abdominopelvic CT protocols used in emergency imaging as well as guidance on the indications for their use. In all cases there will be institutional variation and local departmental guidelines should be followed.

### Non-enhanced CT (NECT)

- The whole abdomen is imaged with contiguous imaging. Ideally it should be acquired during a single breath hold. High-resolution MDCT allows these images to be reviewed in 3D which is particularly helpful in tracing loops of bowel. The images should include the pelvis (to the symphysis pubis) and the domes of both hemi-diaphragms.
- Data is usually reconstructed in 5mm slices. 1–2mm slice reconstruction allows high resolution MPRs to be produced.
- As with thoracic CT, the role of the abdominal NECT is limited in the emergency setting but should be considered for the assessment of haemorrhage prior to the administration of contrast medium, e.g. following trauma or when the patient is being evaluated for a ruptured aneurysm. However, in children and pregnant women, the small potential benefit of such a study must be balanced against the increased radiation exposure and in these cases a single-phase contrast study may be sufficient.

### Contrast enhanced CT (CECT)

Most emergency abdominal CTs are acquired as a single-phase study with a fixed delay of 60–70s for portal phase contrast. However, many variations have been proposed and some suggested protocols are outlined below. As no definitive protocols exist, local guidelines should be followed.

### Oral contrast

- If the patient is nil-by-mouth, ventilated, has a reduced GCS, is at risk of aspiration or may require urgent surgery then oral contrast medium is generally not given. Occasionally, after discussion with the referring team and for a specific indication, it may be given in such circumstances.

- Mix 5ml Gastrografin® in 300ml of water for each dose. *It is important for the radiographer or radiologist to confirm with the nursing staff on the ward that they are familiar with this protocol as administration of neat Gastrograffin® will result in images that are degraded by the dense contrast medium and may be uninterpretable.*
- For a typical abdominal CT, a dose can be given 60min prior to imaging and again at 30min prior to imaging.
- For large bowel studies or assessment of the pelvis, then 4–5 doses of contrast can be given as outlined below.
  - On the evening (8p.m.) 2 days before imaging.
  - 12p.m. on the day before imaging.
  - 8p.m. on the day before imaging.
  - 8a.m. on the day of imaging.
  - A fifth dose may be given just immediately prior to imaging.
  - This protocol is clearly not applicable to emergency imaging.
- Water (without iodinated contrast medium) may be given immediately prior to imaging to distend the stomach to assess both it and the proximal duodenum.

### Rectal contrast

Occasionally rectal contrast can be given prior to abdominal CT. A leak from the sigmoid or rectum (e.g. an anastomotic leak following surgery) can be assessed by giving a small quantity (~100ml) of dilute water-soluble contrast via a Foley catheter prior to imaging.

### Intravenous contrast

- 100–150ml IV contrast at 2–5ml/s.
- Images are usually acquired at a *fixed time* following IV contrast medium administration. Alternatively, images can be *bolus triggered* or a *test bolus* used (see 🕮 p. 61).
- Image acquisition is usually at 60s for a *portal phase* study.
- An *arterial phase* study may also be performed in cases of trauma or for assessment of the liver (as part of a triple-phase hepatic study) at 25s. Arterial assessment of the aorta can be bolus triggered.
- A *pancreatic phase* at 40s is occasionally used to assess pancreatic perfusion in pancreatitis and to identify pancreatic tumours.
- Occasionally a *delayed phase* image (90–120s or sometimes even longer) may be acquired to demonstrate delayed enhancement of an abscess, a slow leak of contrast medium or for assessment of the IVC and iliac veins (e.g. for thrombosis).

## Upper and lower GI contrast studies

The use of such studies is decreasing with the improving resolution of CECT. In the emergency setting, these are primarily used to detect obstruction, perforation or post-operative leak. See Chapter 7 for discussion of upper GI contrast studies.

For a lower GI contrast study, 100–500ml of dilute water-soluble contrast is introduced into the rectum via a Foley catheter while the patient is in the left lateral position. Screening in several anatomical planes is used to identify the leak or level of obstruction. 📖 p. 156 for details.

## Intervention

Once again, arterial phase CT has largely superseded diagnostic arterial angiography for suspected aneurysmal or traumatic leak of the major abdominal vessels as well as for arterial thrombosis. Sagittal MPRs can be used to assess the major proximal branches of the aorta: celiac axis, superior and inferior mesenteric arteries. Diagnostic angiography still has a role in identifying occult bleeding that cannot be identified on upper or lower GI endoscopic examination although MDCT has a similar sensitivity for the detection of gastrointestinal bleeding at rates of 0.5ml/min or more (📖 p. 384).

Nephrostomy is performed to decompress an obstructed renal collecting system in an emergency. US and CT guided drain insertion is an essential part of the emergency management of many patients.

## Other

Endoscopy is used for emergency GI evaluation, particularly in the context of bleeding, but in most centres it is performed by gastroenterologists rather than radiologists. Endoscopic retrograde cholangiopancreatography (ERCP) and magnetic resonance cholangiopancreatography (MRCP) are rarely used in the emergency setting.

---

Checklist for reviewing an abdominal CT to avoid the commonly missed abnormalities.
- Assess the adequacy of the images, e.g. is the opacification sufficient? Has the CT been acquired in all appropriate phases for the abnormality in question.
- Review images on abdominal, liver and bone window settings (📖 Table 4.1 p. 65). Lung window settings can be helpful in identifying free intra-abdominal air.
- Review multiplanar reformatted images. For instance, sagittal images can be useful for assessing the patency of the proximal branches of the abdominal aorta.
- Consider MIP imaging for the assessment of the vasculature.
- Carefully review each organ in turn: liver, spleen, pancreas, kidneys and adrenals.
- Assess soft tissues.
- Trace the large bowel along its length looking for masses, focal narrowing or dilatation. If possible, trace the small bowel.
- Look for stranding in the mesenteric fat—often this may alert the radiologist to the anatomical location of the abnormality.

- In all cases of acute abdominal pain, free intra-abdominal air and fluid must be excluded. Free air will usually be present anteriorly within the abdomen on CT if the patient is in the usual supine position, e.g. adjacent to the falciform ligament; a common error is to miss small focal pockets of free air adjacent to a perforated loop of bowel that has become contained by the surrounding inflammatory response; these pockets may be misinterpreted as a bowel loop. If no obvious abnormality can be identified, pay particular attention to the appendix and try to identify renal calculi.
- In cases where the patient has been referred with suspected renal colic and where no calculus is demonstrated on the unenhanced CT, always try and exclude other causes for the pain (e.g. appendicitis, aortic aneurysm, cholecystitis and pancreatitis) and consider whether a portal phase study may aid the diagnosis.

# Indications for emergency abdominal and pelvic US and CT

The indications for thoracic US and CT imaging in trauma and acute abdominal pain are listed below.

## Traumatic

Many patients will have an AXR on admission to the emergency department. This can be useful in the assessment of fractures and penetrating foreign bodies but is rarely diagnostic.

US can be useful for the following:
- To detect intraperitoneal fluid (either with a departmental US or a FAST study in the emergency department; 📖 p. 69).
- US can be useful in the initial assessment of patients with suspected renal injury *but a negative US does not exclude renal injury.*[2]
- To assess solid organ trauma (i.e. liver, spleen and kidneys) particularly in children or pregnant women in whom radiation dose should be carefully considered. However, US is not only user-dependent but also has a low sensitivity for splenic, GI tract and urological injury.[2]

Intravenous urography (IVU) is occasionally used in some centres but has largely been superseded by CT: its use is mostly limited to unstable patients on their way to theatre or during surgery.

CT is sensitive and specific for major abdominal trauma and is the investigation of choice in most cases.[2] Thoracic, C-spine and head CT should be considered at the same time if appropriate.

## Acute abdominal pain

The portal phase CECT is now the major acute imaging tool for patients presenting with acute abdominal pain. It can be used to identify a wide range of abdominal conditions such as appendicitis, diverticulitis, renal calculi and small bowel obstruction. Furthermore, early abdominopelvic CT for acute abdominal pain may reduce mortality and length of hospital stay and it may also identify unforeseen conditions.[3] The increase in demand for urgent abdominopelvic CT in the context of acute abdominal pain can pose huge challenges for a radiology department. Increasing an out of hours service may mean that staff are unavailable the following day for routine clinical work and this can affect waiting lists and the management of non-urgent patients. Each hospital has therefore to assess its ability to provide on-call imaging and most have drawn up protocols which should be referred to.

There are no formal national or international guidelines for the use of CT in the setting of the acute abdomen. However, when considering which patients are appropriate for urgent abdominopelvic CT the radiologist should consider the following points regarding alternative modalities:
- Only stable patients should be imaged with CT: the unstable patient should either be stabilized before coming to the radiology department or should be taken to the operating theatre.
- Radiographs:
  - Supine AXR may be sufficient to establish a diagnosis of obstruction and may point to an anatomical level.[2]

- Contrast studies:
  - In acute small bowel obstruction, a plain radiograph 4–6hrs after 100ml of oral contrast medium can be a good predictor of resolution.[2]
  - A contrast enema can be used to confirm the diagnosis and level of an obstruction.
- US:
  - Is sensitive for free fluid in perforation.
  - May be used to identify appendicitis if the operator has appropriate training and experience.
  - Is the investigation of choice to demonstrate or to exclude gall-stones and acute cholecystitis.[2]
  - Is the investigation of choice for the female pelvis.
  - Should always be considered first in children, women of reproductive age and pregnant women to avoid radiation exposure.
- Endoscopy:
  - This is the initial investigation for intestinal blood loss from the upper GI tract and colon.[2]
  - Sigmoidoscopy can be used in the assessment of low obstructions identified on AXR.
- CT:
  - The single best investigation when the diagnosis is unknown.
  - High sensitivity for perforation and can identify localized perforations.
  - High sensitivity for renal tract calculi.

As in all aspects of medicine and radiology, do not forget that the request for imaging is not just a piece of paper or an electronic message, it represents a sick patient in need of help. Both the clinician who has requested the imaging, and the radiographers and radiologists performing it, should remember to put the patient's interests first at all times.

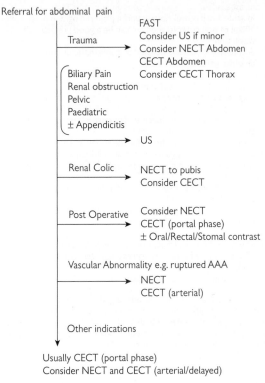

Referral for abdominal pain

Trauma
→
FAST
Consider US if minor
Consider NECT Abdomen
CECT Abdomen
Consider CECT Thorax

Biliary Pain
Renal obstruction
Pelvic
Paediatric
± Appendicitis
→ US

Renal Colic
→
NECT to pubis
Consider CECT

Post Operative
→
Consider NECT
CECT (portal phase)
± Oral/Rectal/Stomal contrast

Vascular Abnormality e.g. ruptured AAA
→
NECT
CECT (arterial)

Other indications
↓
Usually CECT (portal phase)
Consider NECT and CECT (arterial/delayed)

**Fig. 4.5** Suggested protocols for abdominopelvic CT imaging depending on the clinical presentation.

## Further reading

**1.** Grainger and Allison's Diagnostic Radiology: A textbook of Medical Imaging; 4th edition; 2001.

**2.** Making the best use of clinical radiology services: referral guidelines. Royal College of Radiologists 2007.

**3.** Ng CS *et al* (2002) Evaluation of early abdominopelvic computed tomography in patients with acute abdominal pain of unknown cause: prospective randomised study *BMJ* **325**(7377); 1387.

# Postoperative complications

Following surgery, general complications or specific complications related to the operation site may arise. The following presents a list of the more urgent complications, both general and specific, which usually require further imaging.

## General

### Respiratory

*Adult Respiratory Distress Syndrome (ARDS)*

- Acute lung injury occurring in the first 24hrs post-operatively.
- Clinical features: acute dyspnoea, severe hypoxaemia.
- Causes: includes septic or haemorrhagic shock and aspiration.
- Diagnosis:
  - CXR: patchy alveolar infiltrates at 24–48hrs, massive airspace consolidation by 5–7 days, reticular changes after 7 days due to developing fibrosis.
  - CT: consolidation in dependent lung, ground glass infiltrates in non-dependent lung; later, reticular change is seen in an anterior distribution.
- Treatment: intensive supportive care, ventilation.

### Cardiovascular

*Haemorrhagic shock*

- Occurs in the first few hours post-operatively.
- Causes: inadequate haemostasis, may be underlying clotting disorder.
- CT (pre and post IV contrast medium in a portal venous phase)
  - High-density haematoma within pelvis on pre-contrast study
  - Extravasated contrast medium on a delayed study.
- Treatment:
  - Fluid resuscitation, blood transfusion, clotting factors, platelets.
  - Transfemoral angiographic embolisation of bleeding artery.
  - Surgery: haematoma removed, bleeding controlled.

### Deep-vein thrombosis (DVT)

**Table 4.2** Comparison of various imaging techniques for diagnosing DVT

|  | Overall sensitivity (%) | Sensitivity for proximal DVT (%) | Sensitivity for distal DVT (%) | Overall Specificity (%) |
|---|---|---|---|---|
| Compression | 90 | 94 | 57 | 98 |
| Colour Doppler | 82 | 96 | 44 | 93 |
| Duplex | 92 | 97 | 72 | 94 |
| CT venography | 95 | NA | NA | 97 |
| MR venography (time of flight or contrast enhanced) | 92 | NA | NA | 95 |

- Clinical features: calf swelling and pain.
- Occurs in 7–45% of patients postoperatively.
- Risk factors: poor mobilization, sepsis, malignancy, smoking, length of surgery, OCP, HRT.
- Choice of investigations: see Table 4.2.
- Treatment: anticoagulation with subcutaneous low molecular weight heparin for 6 weeks.

### Pulmonary embolism (PE)

- Clinical features: dyspnoea, pleuritic chest pain, haemoptysis <20%, low grade pyrexia, right heart strain.
- 50% occur within first 24 hours, 75% by 72 hours.
- Incidence of fatal PEs postoperatively is 0.2%.
- Accounts for 40% of deaths in gynaecology.
- 75% originate from leg DVT.
- Wells criteria is a validated method of stratifying patients into low, intermediate or high risk, based on risk factors. It is used to determine if imaging investigations are required (See 📖 p. 84).

**Table 4.3** Choice of investigations for PE

|  | Sensitivity (%) | Specificity (%) |
| --- | --- | --- |
| CTPA (multidetector thin collimation)* | 96 | 86 |
| Ventilation/perfusion | 98 | 88 |

- Choice of investigations: see Table 4.3.
  - CT pulmonary angiogram (CTPA) is more accurate than ventilation perfusion scan (V/Q) as it detects PE in V/Q assigned low and intermediate risk groups. Multidetector thin collimation CTPA can detect PEs to the subsegmental level. CTPA may also show an alternative diagnosis for the patient's symptoms.
  - V/Q scan involves a perfusion study with technetium 99m-labelled macroaggregated albumin and a ventilation study with technetium aerosol, xenon gas or krypton.

### Gastrointestinal

*Bowel obstruction*
- Usually small bowel obstruction, due to adhesions.
- Occurs in 0.2–8% of patients after abdominal hysterectomy.
- Presents on the 5th–7th postoperative day and may occur months to years later.
- Clinical features: colicky abdominal pain, abdominal distension, vomiting, constipation.
- Diagnosis:
  - Supine AXR: multiple dilated loops of bowel with no gas in the large bowel (if small bowel obstruction).
  - CT performed with IV contrast in portal venous phase: multiple dilated fluid filled loops of small bowel with transition point identified where collapsed bowel is seen distally.

- Treatment: usually conservative with nasogastric tube (NGT) and IV fluids; occasionally surgery.

### Pseudomembranous colitis

- Cause: Exposure to antibiotics leads to overgrowth of *clostridium difficile* which produces toxins, leading to colitis.
- Typically develops 5–10 days after start of antibiotics.
- Clinical features: bloody diarrhea, pyrexia, abdominal pain and distension.
- Diagnosis:
  - Stool culture; identify toxin in stool
  - AXR: dilated bowel with thumbprinting; if severe can get toxic megacolon with perforation
  - Contrast enema: historical examination which has largely been replaced CT; nodular filling defects seen representing pseudomembranous plaques, haustral thickening and thumbprinting
  - CT performed with IV contrast in a portal venous phase: large bowel wall thickening (low attenuation due to oedema), mucosal enhancement due to hyperaemia, 'target' sign (due to combination of the above two), 'accordion sign' (due to trapping of oral contrast material between haustral folds), pericolonic stranding and ascites
- Treatment: oral metronidazole and vancomycin.
- Rarely need surgical resection.

## Operative site complications

### Haematoma

- Due to intermittent or slow continuous venous bleeding.
- Present by 3rd post-operative day with mass and anaemia.
- Tenderness and pyrexia if it becomes infected.
- Diagnosis: haematoma identified on CT (post intravenous contrast in portal venous phase) or ultrasound.
- Treatment depends on site. For example, a pelvic haematoma:
  - <5cm, treat conservatively.
  - >5cm, consider drainage after haematoma has liquefied (after 5th post-operative day) via a non-image guided approach or using CT/US for guidance.

### Collection/abscess

- Clinical features: pyrexia and pain.
- Usually presents in the 3rd–5th post-operative day.
- Usually polymicrobial in aetiology.
- Diagnosis:
  - Ultrasound demonstrates a complex fluid collection with echogenic flecks due to the presence of gas.
  - CT abdomen/pelvis following oral contrast 60–90 and 30min prior to the study. Performed in the portal venous phase following intravenous contrast medium. A rim-enhancing fluid collection is seen ± pockets of gas.

- Treatment
  - Broad spectrum intravenous antibiotics.
  - May drain spontaneously.
  - May need US/CT guided percutaneous drainage.

## Further reading

1. Droegemueller W (2001) Postoperative counselling and management. In MA Stenchever et al., eds, Comprehensive gynaecology, 4th edn, pp. 771–821. Mosby Inc, St Louis, MI, USA.

2. Goodacre S, Sampson F, Stevenson M et al. (2006). Measurement of the clinical and cost-effectiveness of non-invasive diagnostic testing strategies for deep venous thrombosis. Health Technol Assess 10(15); 1–168.

# Chapter 5

# Respiratory

**Anthony Edey**

# ⑦ Pulmonary thromboembolism

## Epidemiology
- Annual incidence 60–70 cases per 100 000.
- 50% of these develop in hospital or long-term care.

## Aetiology
The majority arise from deep venous clots in the lower limbs. Predisposing factors include immobility, hypercoagulable states (including malignancy), pregnancy, surgery and increasing age.

## Clinical features
The clinical symptoms of PE are non-specific. Especially in severe pulmonary embolism, the abnormalities detected on clinical examination and routine investigations are of limited diagnostic value. Symptoms may range from classical (pleuritic pain associated with dyspnoea and hypoxaemia) to cough and fever. All patients in whom the diagnosis is considered should have an assessment of clinical probability. The British Thoracic Society guidelines (BTSG[1]) recommend use of the Wells Criteria: see Table 5.1.

**Table 5.1** Wells' criteria for assessment of pretest probability for pulmonary embolism

| Criteria | Points | Score range | Interpretation of risk |
|---|---|---|---|
| Suspected DVT | 3.0 | <2 points | Low |
| An alternative diagnosis is less likely than PE | 3.0 | 2–6 points | Moderate |
| Heart rate >100 beats per minute | 1.5 | >6 points | High |
| Immobilization or surgery in the previous four weeks | 1.5 | | |
| Previous DVT or PE | 1.5 | | |
| Hemoptysis | 1.0 | | |
| Malignancy (on treatment, treated in the past 6 months or palliative) | 1.0 | | |

## Imaging
- Imaging for non-massive PE should be performed within 24hrs, and within 1hr for massive PE. Massive PE in clinically unstable patients can be confidently diagnosed using transthoracic echocardiography demonstrating right ventricular enlargement or poor right ventricular function (BTSG).
- Unsuspected PE as an incidental finding on CECT scans may be present in up to 6% of all scans (the incidence is higher in older patients) ∴ on all routine contrast enhanced studies of the thorax the pulmonary arterial tree should be inspected for signs of PE (see Fig. 5.1).[2]

**PIOPED II** (prospective investigation of pulmonary embolism diagnosis)
- 773 patients with an average age of 52 years. 75% were hospitalized from the community.
  - Overall: sensitivity of PE-protocol CT was 83% and specificity 96%, yielding a positive predictive value (PPV) of 86% and a negative predictive value (NPV) of 95%.
  - If low or moderate clinical risk (see above) then CTPA had a 89–96% NPV.
  - If high clinical risk, then the NPV of a normal CTPA was only 60%.

Therefore:
- Additional testing is recommended when clinical probability is inconsistent with test results.

## Radiographs: CXR

No sign is specific, and the sensitivity of the described signs is poor.
- Oligaemia of the lung distal to the occluded vessel (Westermark's Sign); Fig. 5.1
- Linear atelectasis
- Pulmonary infarction may cause consolidation—usually multifocal in the lower zones or a triangular opacity in contact with pleural surface ('Hamptons hump')

## V/Q scan

The Fleischner society position statement[3] summarizes the role of scintigraphy as 'a preferred alternative chest imaging technique for patients who cannot undergo CT angiography, with reduced cost and radiation dose'.
- Indicated, if available, in patients with a normal contemporaneous CXR
- A normal perfusion scan excludes PE with a negative predictive value close to 100%, and as a stand-alone test it is cheap, quick and has a low radiation burden
- High clinical risk and high probability V/Q: 96% PPV
- Unfortunately 75% of V/Q are indeterminate (PIOPED)
- Intermediate V/Q scans require further imaging—i.e. CTPA

## CT pulmonary angiography

### Protocol[4]

MDCT with preferably 16 slices or above. A uniphasic bolus injection of 100ml at 4ml/s (370mg iodine/ml) via an 18G or 20G venous catheter in the antecubital fossa; 20s delay; scan in a caudal to cranial direction; and perform with a single breath hold. An alternative method involves bolus tracking with the region of interest marker set over the central pulmonary vessels and the scanner set to trigger at a preset level of opacification. Departmental practices differ according to experience.

### Image interpretation and quality

- PE-specific (WW 700, WL 100HU), mediastinal (WW 350, WL 40HU) and lung (WW 1500, WL–600HU) windows (see also 📖 p. 65).
- Multiplanar reformats (MPRs) and maximum intensity projections (MIPs) for problem-solving.
- Is the scan adequate? If not, to what anatomical level can the vessels be seen i.e. subsegmental, lobar etc.

- *Motion artefacts*
  - Commonest artefact. Worst at bases.
  - May result in an apparent opacity due to partial voluming. Minimized on MDCT with reduced scan time.
- *Poor opacification*
  - Mean density of acute embolus 33HU, chronic embolus 87HU.
  - A useful rule of thumb is that the minimum required arterial opacification is 200HU, below this level the scan is non-diagnostic. Optimal optimal opacification is achieved with densities of >230HU.
- *Flow artefacts*
  - Transient disruption of enhancement within a vessel due to increased flow of unopacified blood from IVC. Minimized by patient simply holding their breath (not deep inspiration or hyperventilation) thus reducing venous return.
- *Body habitus*
  - Increased image noise. Review study on 2.5mm thick reconstruction to minimize this (note this can reduce sensitivity).

*Findings*

*Direct signs of pulmonary embolism*

- A filling defect within an opacified pulmonary artery. This may completely occlude vessel or have a rim of contrast surrounding the embolus. The latter will appear as a 'tram track' when viewed parallel to the scan plane. Most emboli lyse following an acute episode, but may leave a residual web. Chronic emboli may recanalize and can appear as crescentic thrombi subjacent to the arterial wall.

*Indirect signs of pulmonary embolism*

Presence of the following signs is variable.

- Distal vessel calibre:
  - Vessels distal to embolus may be of reduced calibre
- Infarcts:
  - A characteristic appearance is of a wedge-shaped peripheral focus of consolidation with regional heterogeneous ground-glass opacification (adjacent haemorrhage); Fig. 5.1.
- Mosaic attenuation pattern (chronic thromboembolic disease):
  - Due to heterogeneous perfusion—hypodense regions of lung parenchyma are abnormal and characterized by a relative paucity and reduction in the calibre of vessels, cf. patchy ground-glass in which vessels are of normal calibre and number in hypodense regions.

*Adverse prognostic indicators*

Maximum short axis diameter of right ventricle:left ventricle
Ratio of 1.0 = 5 % risk of death, ratio of 2.3 = 50% risk of death.[5]

## CT venography

- Combining CTPA and CT venography (CTV) of femoral regions increases sensitivity of CTPA (PIOPED). However, this results in a significant increase in radiation. Whilst it may provide a fast 'one-stop-shop' approach to a complete vascular assessment, Doppler evaluation of the lower limbs is probably preferable.[3]

### Pulmonary embolism in pregnancy

- Discussion with senior clinicians/radiologist/medical physicist is advised.
- Leg doppler advised for DVT. If positive patient will probably require anticoagulation regardless and radiation may be avoided.
- CTPA exposes the foetus to a lower dose of radiation than V/Q scanning (CTPA foetal dose in early pregnancy 3.3–20.2μGy, V/Q 740 μGy; in late pregnancy CTPA 51–130 μGy, V/Q 640 μGy).[6]
- CTPA exposes mother (including breasts which during lactation are more vulnerable to radiation) to a higher dose than V/Q.
- If the CXR is normal, a perfusion scan alone is probably the first line investigation as it avoids administration of iodinated contrast media and reduces absorbed dose.[3]
- A half dose Q scan will further decrease the radiation burden. The patient spends twice as long in image acquisition in order to reach an adequate number of counts in the image.
- Although no consensus is available on the best imaging strategies, the Royal College of Obstetricians and Gynaecologists (RCOG, UK) advises that if a CXR and Doppler US are normal, a V/Q (or perfusion only scan) or CTPA should be performed depending on local availability and following discussion with a radiologist; women should be advised that V/Q carries a slightly increased risk of childhood cancer compared with CTPA (1/280 000 versus less than 1/1 000 000) but carries a lower risk of maternal breast cancer (lifetime risk increased by up to 13.6% with CTPA, background risk of 1/200 for study population).[7]

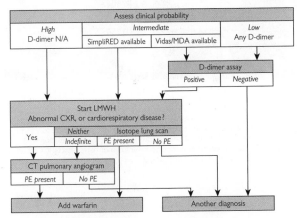

**Fig. 5.1** BTS flowchart for the management of suspected (non-massive) pulmonary embolism where scintigraphy is available on site (reproduced from reference 1). LMWH, low molecular weight heparin.
D-dimer tests:
- SimpliRED: red cell agglutination test.
- Vidas: Entyme-Linked ImmunoSorbent Assay (ELISA).
- MDA: latex D-dimer test.

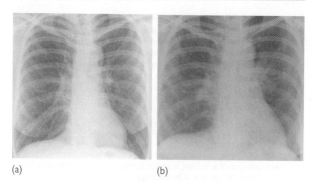

**Fig. 5.2** (a) Normal PA radiograph performed as part of routine pre-operative assessment for total hip replacement. (b) Post-operatively the patient became haemodynamically unstable and desaturated. AP radiograph shows pruning of the pulmonary vasculature (Westermark's sign) and prominence of the perihilar regions. A large saddle-embolus was confirmed on CTPA.

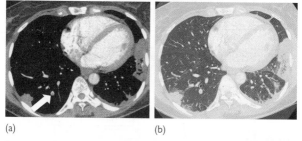

**Fig. 5.3** (a) Standard CECT with mediastinal window settings; there was no suspicion of a PE clinically therefore CTPA was not performed. Note the filling defect in the right posterior basal segmental pulmonary artery (arrow). (b) Lung window settings at the same level shows bilateral peripheral triangular foci of consolidation with regional ground-glass opacification consistent with haemorrhagic infarcts. *It is important to look for incidental emboli on all thoracic CECTs.*

## Further reading

**1.** British Thoracic Society Standards of Care Committee Pulmonary Embolism Guideline Development Group (2003) British Thoracic Society guidelines for the treatment of suspected acute pulmonary embolism. *Thorax* **58**; 470–84.

**2.** Ritchie G, McGurk S, McCreath C et al. (2007) Prospective evaluation of unsuspected pulmonary embolism on contrast-enhanced multidetector CT (MDCT) scanning. *Thorax* **62**; 536–40.

**3.** Remy-Jardin M, Pistolesi M, Goodman LR et al. (2007) Management of suspected acute pulmonary embolism in the era of CT angiography: a statement from the Fletcher Society. *Radiology* **245**; 315–29. **Read this if none of the other references.**

**4.** Wittram C(2007) How I do it: CT pulmonary angiography. *AJR* **188**: 1255–61. **A practical guide to CTPA.**

**5.** Ghuysen A, Ghaye B, Willems V et al. (2005) Computed tomographic pulmonary angiography and prognostic significance in patients with acute pulmonary embolism. *Thorax* **60**; 956–61.

**6.** Groves AM, Yates SJ, Win T et al. (2006) CT pulmonary angiography versus ventilation–perfusion scintigraphy in pregnancy: implications from a UK survey of doctors' knowledge exposure. *Radiology* **240(3)**; 765–70.

**7.** RCOG (2007) *Thromboembolic Disease in Pregnancy and the Peurperium: Acute Management.* Greentop Guideline 28, available at http://www.rcog.org.uk/index.asp?PageID=533.

## :⚙: **Pneumothorax**

### Clinical features

- Ranges in presentation depending on cause. Pleuritic chest pain and breathlessness are common. In the worst case, a tension pneumothorax may cause cardiac arrest (pulseless electrical activity) as a result of a restrictive ventilatory defect and respiratory failure. In trauma, detection is particularly important even if the pneumothorax is small, as mechanical ventilation or general anaesthesia may cause a significant increase in size.

### Aetiology

- Spontaneous: $1°$ or $2°$ to pre-existing lung disease. $1°$ spontaneous is common in asthenic young men and due to a ruptured pleural bleb.
- Traumatic: including iatrogenic.
- Tension pneumothorax occurs when the intrapleural pressure in the affected hemithorax becomes positive and most commonly is due to trauma (when a tear in the pleural surface acts as a one-way valve) but can also be present in ventilated patients.

### Imaging

#### Radiographs

*Erect CXR*

- Air rises in the pleural cavity separating the visceral pleura from the chest wall. A sharply defined curvilinear line with no lung markings peripherally is seen.
- False positives:
  - Skin folds extend beyond the chest and have a broad edge which is well defined laterally but fades medially.
  - Bullae: the inner margin is concave to the chest wall, not convex and does not conform to the shape of the costophrenic angle.
- Depression of the ipsilateral hemidiaphragm is the most sensitive sign of tension and, particularly in ventilated patients, is more sensitive than contralateral mediastinal shift (airway pressure remains positive).

*Supine CXR*

- Sensitivity 50–70% (i.e. significantly less than an erect radiograph).
- If doubt remains, a lateral decubitus film with the suspected side up may be helpful for confirmation.
- Free air rises to the anterior and anteromedial thorax ∴ seen as hypochondrial lucency, a deep lateral costophrenic sulcus and, particularly in infants, increased visibility of the adjacent mediastinal margin.

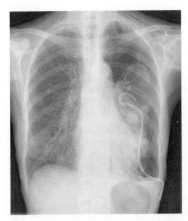

**Fig. 5.4** PA erect chest radiograph showing a large left pneumothorax with an intercostal chest drain in place. The visceral pleural margin is a crisp radio-opaque line. Peripheral to the pleural edge, the thorax is avascular.

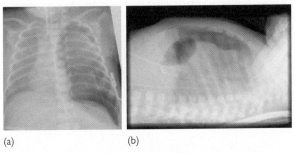

(a)                                    (b)

**Fig. 5.5** (a) Supine mobile radiograph in an intubated infant with a large left-sided pneumothorax. Note the depression of the left hemidiaphragm ('deep sulcus') and contralateral mediastinal shift indicating tension. The clinical team needs to be contacted immediately to alert them to these potentially life-threatening findings. (b) Horizontal beam lateral radiograph of a different infant. The distribution of air in the pleural space is clearly demonstrated. Note the anterior costophrenic sulcus is pushed inferiorly. This is a useful technique, particularly in infants, for confirming the presence of a supine pneumothorax.

*Ultrasound*

*Protocol*

Curvilinear probe 3.5–5MHz. Highly user-dependent.

*Findings*

Normally the visceral pleura is visible 'gliding' under the parietal pleura, if a pneumothorax is present this is not seen and there is extensive reverberation artefact beneath the parietal pleura.

## CT

*Protocol*

Standard departmental protocol with or without IV contrast medium.

*Findings*

The gold standard imaging tool. Remember the distribution of free thoracic air for supine imaging, small pneumothoraces will be visible anteromedially.

## Complications

- Pleural fluid which is seen in trauma and with primary spontaneous cases. A haemopneumothorax is commonly present.
- Re-expansion oedema: follows chest drain placement. May be unilateral or bilateral. 20% mortality.

## Management

Tension pneumothorax: give maximum available inspired oxygen. Insert the largest peripheral venous cannula available (at least 18G) into the second intercostal space in the mid-clavicular line on the affected side. This should achieve immediate relief. Call for urgent medical support.

## Further reading

**1.** Beckh S, Böleskei Pl and Lessnau KD (2002) Real-time chest ultrasonography: a comprehensive review for the pulmonologist. *Chest* **122**; 1759–73.

**2.** Tocino IM, Miller MH, Frederick PR *et al.* (1984) CT detection of occult pneumothorax in head trauma. *AJR* **143**; 987–90.

**3.** Hansell DM, Armstrong P, Lynch DA and Page McAdams H (2004) *Imaging Diseases of the Chest*, 4th edn. Mosby.

## ⑦ Pneumonia

### Clinical features

- Presentation ranges from productive cough with fever to generalized sepsis and confusion. It may be life-threatening in vulnerable groups (e.g. the elderly, those with underlying cardiac or lung pathology).
- Knowledge of the underlying immune status is vital.

### Consolidation

- Consolidation is caused by displacement of alveolar air by pus, blood, fluid, or cancer (and is a subdivision of the broader term 'airspace opacification').
- Persistent consolidation despite antibiotic therapy is worrying—both lymphoma and bronchoalveolar cell carcinoma may present in this way.
- Multifocal consolidation should always trigger three diagnostic possibilities: aspiration, unusual organisms such as tuberculosis (TB) or mycoplasma pneumonia (or in the context of immunocompromise, opportunistic infections).
- CT and CXR: poorly defined opacity (except when it abuts a fissure) which obscures vessels and may contain air bronchograms. It may start as acinar nodules measuring 0.5–1cm in diameter which then coalesce.

### Patterns of infection

- None is diagnostic of an organism and microbiological confirmation is required.
- Below are examples of the basic patterns of infection with the typical infectious agents associated with the pattern.

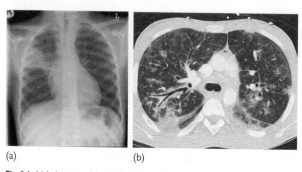

(a)                              (b)

**Fig. 5.6** (a) Lobar consolidation. The classical presentation of *Streptococcus pneumoniae*. Consolidation is limited by pleural boundaries. (b) Bronchopneumonia. Patchy, multifocal, heterogeneous consolidation, with bronchial wall thickening. Commonly seen with *Mycoplasma pneumoniae, S. aureus, H. influenzae*.

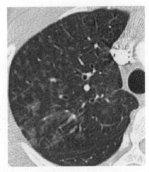

**Fig 5.7** Tree-in-bud. Soft centrilobular opacities with extension into peripheral branching opacities (plugged centrilobular bronchioles). This indicates an exudative bronchiolitis most commonly as a result of infection. Seen in TB, atypical mycobacterial infections, *M. pneumoniae*, aspiration, *H. influenzae*, RSV and many other infections.

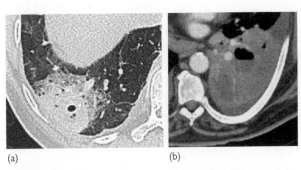

(a)                              (b)

**Fig 5.8** Cavitation/abscess formation: *S. aureus*, Klebsiella, TB, *Pseudomonas aeruginosa*, fungal infections.

## Infection in the immunocompromised patient

- Focal consolidation is most likely to be due to bacterial infection.
- Nodules are likely to be due to mycobacterial infection or fungus.
- A diffuse or interstitial pattern raises the possibility of PCP or viral infections.

### HIV: the numbers game

CD4 count determines the probable causative organism:
- CD4 >200 × 10⁶ cells/l: bacterial pneumonia, TB (reinfection).
- CD4 50–200 × 10⁶ cells/l: bacterial pneumonia, TB (primary), pneumocystis pneumonia (PCP), fungal infections.

- CD4 <50 x $10^6$ cells/l: bacterial pneumonia, atypical appearances of TB, PCP, fungal infections, mycobacterium avium complex (MAC), cytomegalovirus (CMV).

NB PCP is caused by the fungus, *Pneumocystis jiroveci* (in honour of the Czech parasitologist Otto Jírovec, one of the first researchers to describe Pneumocystis infection in humans) not, as originally thought, a protozoan.[1]

### Bone marrow transplants (BMT)

*Neutropenic phase complications (0 to 30 days post-BMT)*

- Bacterial: similar range of appearances as in immunocompetent patients.
- Angioinvasive aspergillosis: nodules with halo of ground glass.
- Candida: focal or multifocal consolidation.

*Early phase (31 to 100 days post-BMT)*

- Viral: especially CMV, which may have non-specific appearance including multifocal consolidation and centrilobular nodules.

### Solid organ transplants

Broadly similar pattern of infection to BMT reflecting severity of immune-suppression but also consider PCP between 1 and 6 months.

### Further reading

**1.** *J Eukaryot Microbiol* 2001; **48**(suppl); 1S–204S. Entire supplement.

# ⑦ **Pleural effusion**

## Definition and aetiology

- Historically an exudate has been defined as pleural fluid with a protein content of >30g/L, whilst a transudate contains <30g/L.
- Aspirates between 25–35g/L are relatively non-specific and the following is used to diagnose an exudative effusion in this context:
  - Pleural fluid protein divided by serum protein >0.5 or
  - Pleural fluid LDH divided by serum LDH >0.6 or
  - Pleural fluid LDH >2/3rds the upper limits of normal serum LDH.

|  | Transudates | Exudates |
|---|---|---|
| Common | Left venticular failure | Malignancy |
|  | Liver cirrhosis | Parapneumonic effusion |
|  | Hypoalbuminaemia |  |
|  | Peritoneal dialysis |  |
| Uncommon | Hypothyroidism | Pulmonary infarction |
|  | Nephrotic syndrom | Rheumatoid arthritis |
|  | Mitral stenosis | Pancreatitis |
|  | Pulmonary embolism | Post myocardial infarct |

## Clinical features

- Effusions may cause significant respiratory compromise, or be a marker of underlying disease.

## Imaging

### Chest radiographs

*Erect CXR*

- The typical radiographic appearance is of a curved meniscus.
- Estimating the volume: 150mls blunts the costophrenic angle; 200mls renders meniscus visible; 500mls obscures the hemidiaphragm.
- A large effusion causes mediastinal shift, cf. lung atelectasis.
- Subpulmonic effusions conceal a large volume of fluid and causes:
  - Apparent elevation of the hemidiaphragm
  - Lateral peaking of the pseudo-diaphragm
  - Blunting of the lateral costophrenic sulcus.
- Be aware of loculated fluid which may be seen as a biconvex pleurally based opacity, or lie in the fissure causing a 'psuedotumour'.

*Supine CXR*

- Fluid tracks posteriorly and results in a veil-like opacity with preserved vascular markings and loss of clarity of the ipsilateral hemidiaphragm.

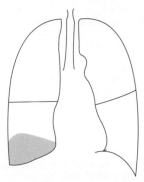

**Fig. 5.9** Diagrammatic representation of a right subpulmonic effusion. The shaded area represents fluid and is easily mistaken for the diaphragm. Note that the apex of the fluid is more lateral than the normal diaphragmatic dome. The diaphragm itself is not visible and is often bowed inferiorly by the volume of fluid.

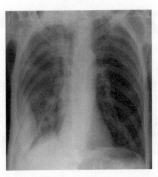

**Fig. 5.10** PA erect CXR showing a pleural lesion (well defined medially, poorly defined laterally) with no underlying rib destruction in the right base. If there is clinical doubt an ultrasound may be of value to confirm that the abnormality is a loculated pleural effusion, as was the case here.

### US
Protocol
- Detection of small effusions is optimized by lying the patient supine for >10 min prior to study and then positioning in a lateral decubitus position—affected side up—scan posteriorly from the midline outwards.
- 3.5–5MHz curvilinear probe.

*Findings*
- Anechoic/hypoechoic effusions may be exudates or transudates.
- However, typically exudates contain septae and may show pleural thickening. Uniformly hyperechoic fluid is likely to be due empyema or haemothorax.
- Hyperechoic fluid may be distinguished from solid lesions by the presence of swirling in the fluid on respiration, and the presence of Doppler signal during respiration.

## CT

*Protocol*
- Standard chest CT protocol.

*Findings*
- A hypodense crescent in the dependent pleural space. Symmetrical effusions are often the result of cardiac dysfunction.
- Signs suggestive of an inflammatory or infective effusion include loculation, the presence of parenchymal bands in the underlying lung and thickening of the extrapleural fat (Fig. 5.11).
- Parietal and visceral pleural thickening with enhancement of the visceral pleura may be a feature of an empyema.

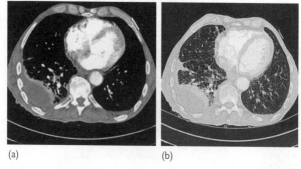

(a)                                        (b)

**Fig. 5.11** (a) Mediastinal window settings: a loculated right basal pleural effusion is shown with thickened, enhancing visceral pleura visible. (b) Lung window settings: there are numerous parenchymal bands in the underlying lung. The CT appearances are suggestive of an empyema and this was confirmed on aspiration. The patient was referred to the cardiothoracic surgeons and had a large bore chest drain inserted.

## Complications

- Parapneumonic effusions are common (seen in about 40% of pneumonias). Initially, parapneumonic effusions are sterile exudates. If untreated then bacterial infiltration of the pleural space from contiguous pneumonia leads to a fibropurulent collection. Eventually, fibroblastic activity results in encasement of the lung by a thick membrane ('pleural peel') which destroys the lung function.

- Differentiation of a simple parapneumonic effusion and an organizing empyema is impossible on radiological grounds (although the imaging characteristics previously mentioned may be of value). Early diagnostic aspiration is vital to pre-empt the development of a fibropurulent collection which is difficult to treat conservatively and may require surgical intervention.
- Passive atelectasis is an almost invariable feature associated with pleural effusion in patients with normal lungs. Its absence suggests that the lungs are 'stiff'.

**Table 5.1** Staging and biochemistry of parapneumonic effusions

| Stage | Macroscopic appearance | Pleural fluid characteristics | Comments |
|---|---|---|---|
| Simple parapneumonic | Clear fluid | pH >7.2 | Normally resolves with antibiotics alone |
| | | LDH <1000 | Drain if required on symptomatic grounds |
| Complicated parapneumonic | Clear fluid cloudy/turbid | pH <7.2 LDH >1000 Glucose <2.2mmol/L | Requires chest tube drainage |
| | | May be positive on gram stain/culture | |
| Empyema | Frank pus | May be positive on gram stain/culture | Requires chest tube drainage |
| | | No additional biochemical tests necessary on pleural fluid | |

Adapted from Journal of Postgraduate Medicine.

**Further reading**

1. Maskell NA and Butland RJA (2003) BTS guidelines for the investigation of a unilateral pleural effusion in adults. *Thorax* **58**; 8–17.

2. Kearney SE, Davies CW, Davies RJ et al. (2000) Computed tomography and ultrasound in parapneumonic effusions and empyema. *Clinical Radiology* **55**; 542–7.

3. Lipscomb DJ, Flower CD and Hadfield JW (1981) Ultrasound of the pleura: an assessment of its clinical value. *Clinical Radiology* **32**; 289–90.

4. Medford A and Maskell N (2005) Pleural effusion. *Postgrad Med J* **81**; 702–10.

## ☢☣ Chest trauma

### Clinical features

Imaging plays a key role in the management of body trauma outlined in the ATLS protocols. However, definitive (usually surgical) intervention should not be delayed by unnecessary imaging. To prevent this, discussion between the radiologist and the trauma team leader should precede further tests after the secondary survey is complete.

### Imaging

#### Mobile CXR

A standard component of the ATLS 'trauma series'.

#### CECT

- Standard departmental CECT.
- Consider CT aortography (☐ p. 114).

Review images on mediastinal, bone and lung window settings, with a high resolution filter for the latter two. Three-dimensional reformatting is vital in assessing skeletal and mediastinal injuries.

### Thoracic cage injury

#### Rib fractures

- Fractures of any of the first 3 ribs posteriorly is an indicator of high velocity trauma. Consider brachial plexus or subclavian vascular injuries with upper rib fractures. Lower thoracic fractures should raise the possibility of abdominal organ injury.
- A flail segment consists of at least 2 fractures on each of 3 or more consecutive ribs. This results in paradoxical chest wall movements predisposing the patient to atelectasis and pneumonia; and may require surgical stabilization or intubation—it should therefore be specifically reported to the clinical team.

#### Sternal injuries

Typically fractures are of the manubrium or body and are seen in the context of deceleration injuries (e.g. impact of driver with steering wheel) ∴ may be associated with injury to the aorta and great vessels. May be visible on CXR. 3D reformats of CT are very helpful.

#### Spinal injuries
☐ p. 262.

### Pleural trauma

#### Pneumothorax
☐ p. 90.

#### Haemothorax
CXR

- The plain film findings are the same as for a pleural effusion (☐ p. 98). Rapid enlargement on serial radiographs suggests active arterial bleeding.

*CT*
- On CT, haemothorax has a density of between 35 and 70HU. Occasionally an active bleeding point may be visible on CECT as a non-anatomical high density (within 10HU of the density of an adjacent vessel) in the fluid.

## Lung trauma

### Contusions

The most common lung injury following blunt chest trauma. Damage to the lung parenchyma results in blood in the alveolar and interstitial spaces. Haemorrhage is greatest over the first 24hrs following injury. Contusions tend to have cleared by about 7 days. Persistence of the opacities beyond this time suggests acute respiratory distress (ARDS), pulmonary oedema or infection.

*CXR and CT*
- CT is much more sensitive than plain radiographs.
- Focal or diffuse ill-defined ground-glass opacities which extend across lobar boundaries (cf. pneumonia or aspiration pneumonitis).
- 1–2mm subpleural sparing may be present.
- The extent of contusion has been found to be an indicator of the likelihood of developing ARDS.

### Lung laceration

Disruption of the lung architecture by trauma results in parenchymal cysts. Resolution takes weeks or months. They may be complicated by abscess formation, bronchopleural fistulation (due to communication between the cyst and pleural surface or an adjacent bronchiole) or progressive enlargement (due to a ball-and-valve mechanism which may result in compression of adjacent lung).

*CXR and CT*
- CT is much more sensitive than plain radiographs.
- Lesions may be masked by overlying contusion over the first 48–72hrs.
- Ovoid lung cysts, which may or may not contain fluid, and may be solitary or multiple.

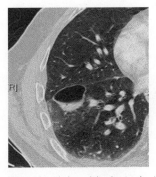

**Fig. 5.12** A lung laceration in the right lower lobe abutting the right oblique fissure is visible with an air/fluid level. The surrounding ground-glass opacity represents resolving contusion. (Image supplied by Dr Sujal Desai.)

### Mediastinal injury (non-vascular)

#### Tracheobronchial injury

Relatively uncommon (<5% of blunt chest trauma) and may by due to penetrating injuries (70%), and blunt trauma (30%). Penetrating injuries commonly involve the cervical trachea. The majority of injuries due to blunt trauma occur within 2.5cm of the carina: the right main bronchus tends to be injured more than the left. The diagnosis is often overlooked both clinically and radiologically.

#### Imaging

- Direct signs may be visible on 3D CT reformats as tracheal deformity or a wall defect.
- Indirect signs include persistent pneumomediastinum or pneumo-thorax despite appropriate treatment (resulting from an air leak) and should raise the diagnostic possibility. Other useful signs are deviation of the endotracheal tube (ETT) from its expected course, and focal herniation of the ETT balloon through a wall defect.

### Oesophageal injury

- 📖 p. 180.

### Further reading

1. Miller LA (2006) Chest wall, lung, and pleural space tauma. *Radiol Clin North Am* **44(2)**; 213–24.

# Line and tube positioning

## Endotracheal tubes

### Positioning

- Approximately 10% are misplaced. The ideal location is mid-tracheal. The tip may move by up to 2cm on neck flexion and extension ∴ the minimum safe distance from the carina is 2cm (if the carina is not visible then assume that it lies at the T4/5 vertebral interspace).

### Complications

- Placement in the right main bronchus may lead to collapse of the left lung, if it extends to the bronchus intermedius the right upper lobe may also collapse.
- Oesophageal placement may cause hypoventilation, with gaseous distension of the stomach and reflux.

## Central venous catheters

### Positioning

- Central venous catheters should ideally lie between the caudal SVC and superior aspect of the right atrium.[1]

### Complications

- Placement in the right atrium may lead to arrhythmias or cardiac perforation, whilst incorrect positioning in the internal jugular or contralateral subclavian increases the risk of thrombus formation or vessel damage.
- Pneumothorax is particularly common in subclavian catheterization, and may be found as a complication in about 5% of all central line placement.

## Swan–Ganz catheters (pulmonary capillary wedge pressure monitors)

### Positioning

- Allows accurate assessment of patient's fluid volume status, and distinction between cardiac and non-cardiac pulmonary oedema.
- The tip should lie in the pulmonary trunk or very proximal main pulmonary arteries—i.e. within the mediastinal shadow.

### Complications

- Placement in the lobar pulmonary vasculature may result in pulmonary infarction or vessel rupture.

## Nasogastric tubes

### Positioning

- Below the diaphragm in the region of the gastric fundus.

### Complications

- Intubation of the bronchi may lead to severe pneumonia, atelectasis or, rarely, pneumothorax. Oesophageal or gastro-oesophageal junction placement predisposes to aspiration.

## Further reading

**1.** Cadman A, Lawrence JA, Fitzsimmons L et al. (2004) To clot or not to clot? That is the question in central venous catheters. Clin Radiol **59**; 349–55.

# ⊙ **Foreign body inhalation**

### Epidemiology and aetiology

- Most commonly seen in children aged under 3yrs.
- Nuts are the commonest inhaled foreign body (FB).
- In the context of trauma teeth may be aspirated.

### Clinical features

- The event may be asymptomatic or, more commonly, result in an episode of wheezing or cough. However, if the object is large enough to obstruct the trachea, then asphyxia and death may occur.
- Up to the age of 15, aspiration is equally common on the left and right; in older patients the right side is more commonly affected (the bronchus intermedius is more vertically orientated than the left lower lobe bronchus and therefore forms the path of least resistance).

### Imaging

#### CXR

- >80% of FBs are radiolucent.
- In acute aspiration, the FB can act as a ball-valve resulting in distal air trapping. This causes hyperlucency of the obstructed segment or lobe, with localized reduction in the visible pulmonary vessels.
- On inspiration the mediastinum is central, but on an expiratory radiograph there may be contralateral midline shift ∴ the inspiratory radiograph may be entirely normal.

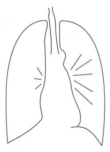

**Fig. 5.13** Diagrammatic representation of aspiration of a foreign body in the right main bronchus. The right hemidiaphragm is flattened and there is shift of the trachea to the left in keeping with air-trapping. There has been a marked reduction in the vascularity (indicated by lines) in the poorly ventilated right lung and compensatory hyperperfusion with prominence of the vasculature in the left lung.

- A lateral decubitus view (affected side down) or fluoroscopy may be useful—persistent hyperexpansion in the dependent lung confirms the presence of obstruction.
- The commonest complications are pneumonia and atelectasis. Chronic retention of the foreign body may result in bronchiectasis.
- In 2% of cases pneumomediastinum or a pneumothorax may occur.

## CT
- CT features mirror the plain radiographic findings

## Differential diagnosis (hyperlucent lung)
- Radiographic technique
- Chest wall asymmetry
- Macleod syndrome
- Bronchial obstruction due to other causes

## Management
- Bronchoscopy

## Further reading
1. Hansell DM, Armstrong P, Lynch D and page McAdams H (2004) *Imaging of Diseases of the Chest*, 4th edn. Mosby.

2. Harris J and Harris W (1999) *The Radiology of Emergency Medicine*; revised 4th edn. Lippincott Williams and Wilkins.

# Acute lung injury and ARDS

Definition and aetiology

- Acute lung injury (ALI) is defined as acute respiratory symptoms and radiographic infiltrates but no evidence of left heart failure with a $PaO_2/FiO_2$ >300.
- Acute respiratory distress syndrome (ARDS) is defined as acute respiratory symptoms and radiographic infiltrates but no evidence of left heart failure with a $PaO_2/FiO_2$ >200.
- ARDS may be due to direct lung injury (pulmonary ARDS) or indirect lung injury (extrapulmonary ARDS). Common aetiologies are listed below:

| Pulmonary ARDS | Extrapulmonary ARDS |
| --- | --- |
| Aspiration | Systemic sepsis |
| Pulmonary infection | Severe non-thoracic trauma |
| Near drowning | Hypertransfusion |
| Toxic fume inhalation | Cardiopulmonary bypass |
| Lung contusion | |

Clinical features

- Respiratory distress with an appropriate inciting event.
- Extra-pulmonary and pulmonary ARDS respond in different ways to mechanical ventilation. Lung compliance is lower in pulmonary ARDS than extrapulmonary ARDS and is further reduced by increasing positive end expiratory pressures which is detrimental to outcome. The converse is true for extrapulmonary ARDS ∴ the distinction on radiological/clinical grounds is important.

Imaging

CXR

- During the 1st 24hrs, the CXR may be normal in extrapulmonary ARDS.
- The first signs are of widespread ground glass opacification which progresses to widespread airspace opacification over the next 36hrs.
- NB bilateral airspace opacification is a non-specific finding—*hydrostatic pulmonary oedema may be indistinguishable.*
- The appearance tends to then remain static for a variable period of time.

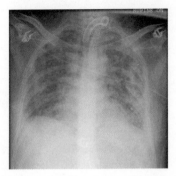

**Fig. 5.14** A typical appearance of ARDS (in this instance pulmonary) with bilateral airspace opacification. Note bilateral chest drains, tracheostomy and NG tube. (Image supplied by Dr Sujal Desai.)

### CT chest

- The typical appearance is of heterogeneous ground-glass opacification with a gradient of density—the dependent regions are more densely opacified than the non-dependent lung. Pulmonary ARDS may have additional non-dependent parenchymal opacities and other 'atypical' features such as cysts. This distinction is useful but not entirely reliable.

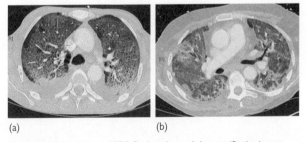

(a)          (b)

**Fig. 5.15** (a) Extrapulmonary ARDS. Graduated ground-glass opacification is seen throughout the lungs, increasing in density in the dependent lungs. Note that underlying centrilobular emphysema is modifying the appearance in parts. (b) Pulmonary ARDS. An atypical appearance of ARDS with multifocal non-dependent opacities which may suggest direct lung injury as the aetiological cause. (Images supplied by Dr Sujal Desai.)

### Further reading

**1.** Desai SR, Wells AU, Suntharalingam G et al. (2001) Acute respiratory distress syndrome caused by pulmonary and extrapulmonary injury: a comparative CT study. *Radiology* **218**; 689–93.

**2.** Desai SR (2002) Acute respiratory distress syndrome: imaging of the injured lung. *Clinical Radiology* **57**; 8–17.

# Cardiovascular

Bobby Agrawal

# ⊕ Aortic dissection

A spontaneous longitudinal split in the media of the aortic wall.

## Aetiology and epidemiology

The pathogenesis is unclear. The following are risk factors:
- Long-standing hypertension
- Marfan's syndrome, Ehlers–Danlos syndrome
- Bicuspid aortic valve
- Pregnancy
- Trauma, usually due to sudden deceleration injuries from motor vehicle accidents
- Cardiac catheterization
- Racial differences: more common in Afro-Caribbeans than in Asians
- M:F 3:1; peak at 50–65 years

## Clinical features

- Symptoms include:
  - sudden onset of tearing interscapular pain
  - severe chest pain
  - stroke-like presentations
- Signs include:
  - hypotension
  - murmur of aortic regurgitation

## Classification

DeBakey I:             Ascending aorta and proximal arch
DeBakey II:          Ascending aorta only
DeBakey III:         Descending aorta only
Stanford Type A:   Ascending aorta and proximal arch
Stanford Type B:   Descending aorta only

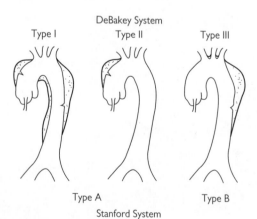

Fig. 6.1 The DeBakey and Stanford classification systems for dissection.

## Imaging

### Radiographs

This is of limited use as a first-line investigation but when performed may show a widened mediastinum (>8cm on PA CXR). This should always be compared to previous films when available. Other suggestive signs are:

- medial deviation of aortic calcification by haematoma
- tracheal displacement to the right
- pleural and/or pericardial effusion
- left apical cap i.e. opacification of the lung apex
- lateral displacement of the oesophagus (as seen with an NG tube)

### US

Transoesophageal echo has a high sensitivity and specificity.

### CT

#### Protocol

NECT of the chest to look for high density intramural haematoma.
CECT: Bolus tracking or triggering can be used. Arterial phase imaging through the chest and abdomen to the aortic bifurcation to assess extent of dissection and involvement of major branches. If available, ECG-gating should be used to help to reduce the number of false-positive studies secondary to aortic root motion. ECG-gating may also help to identify involvement of the coronary arteries and will allow a full assessment of the coronaries prior to surgical intervention.

#### Findings

- Aortic intramural haematoma.
- Intimal flap separating the two lumens; usually the true lumen lined by intima is *smaller* and the false lumen lined by media is *larger*.
- Pleural or pericardial effusions (📖 p. 98 and p 140) which may be high in HU attenuation if haemorrhagic.
- Dissection flaps extending into the major arterial branches; assess for ischaemic thrombosis of the organs these vessels supply.
- Aortic motion in non-ECG gated studies may make evaluation of coronary artery involvement difficult.

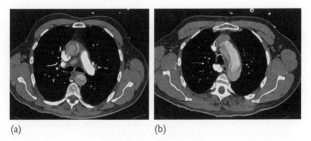

(a)                    (b)

**Fig. 6.2** Two axial CECT images showing a Stanford Type A dissection at the level of the carina (a) and the aortic arch (b). The true lumen is smaller and denser than the false lumen.

*False negatives*
- Poor contrast medium opacification.
- Thrombosed lumen wrongly identified as a mural haematoma in an aneurysm.

*False positives*
- Motion and beam hardening artefacts.
- Mural thrombus in a fusiform aneurysm.

## Angiography

The role of catheter angiography for the diagnosis of aortic dissection is confined to difficult cases where diagnosis is uncertain.

## MRI

Plays little role in the assessment of the acute aortic dissection. It is, however, very useful for follow-up of chronic dissection and following surgical treatment.

## Management

- Stanford type A and DeBakey I or II: surgical management.
- Stanford type B and DeBakey III: medical therapy, i.e. blood pressure control. Endovascular stenting has an emerging role in the management of type B dissection.

## Complications

- Retrograde dissection (Stanford A) leading to pericardial effusion, coronary artery dissection and aortic regurgitation.
- Occlusion of aortic branches, especially those arising from the false lumen.
- Rupture of the aorta.

## Further reading

**1.** Macura J, Corl FM, Fishman EK *et al.* (2003) Pathogenesis in acute aortic syndromes: aortic aneurysm leak and rupture and traumatic aortic resection. *AJR* **181**; 303–7.

**2.** Yu T, Zhu X, Tang L *et al.* (2007) Review of CT angiography of aorta. *Radiol Clin N Am* **45**: 461–83.

# Thoracic aortic aneurysm

Aneurysmal dilatation of the ascending thoracic aorta, aortic arch and/or descending thoracic aorta. Defined as diffuse or focal dilatation by more than 50% of the normal diameter.

## Clinical features

- May be asymptomatic
- Symptoms related to vascular compromise
- Aortic regurgitation from dilatation of the aortic root
- Thromboembolism
- Local mass effect
- SVC obstruction
- Tracheal or main stem bronchus compression
- Oesophageal compression

## Imaging

### Radiographs

*Findings*

- Widening of the mediastinal silhouette: >8cm on a PA radiograph
- Enlargement of the aortic knuckle
- Displacement of the trachea from the midline

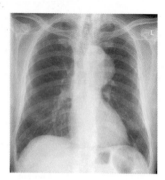

**Fig. 6.3** CXR demonstrating a thoracic aortic aneurysm.

### US

Transoesophageal echo (TOE) is accurate in the detection of aortic valve disease, ascending aortic aneurysm and aortic dissection as well as evaluation of cardiac structure and function. Whilst the majority of patients will undergo examination with CT, TOE has a role to play and can accurately differentiate between ascending and descending aortic dissection.

## CT

Both CT and MRI are the most commonly used techniques for assessment of aortic disease, both before and after surgical intervention. CT is the main imaging modality in the acute setting.

### Protocol

See aortic dissection protocol (📖 p 115).

### Findings

CECT examination of the chest defines the anatomy of the aorta in its entirety. If the study is ECG-gated, then excellent detail of the mobile ascending aorta and aortic root can be obtained which enhances surgically planning.

## MRI

MRI provides both anatomical and functional data. It can measure the degree of aortic valve regurgitation and differential flow in the true and false lumens of a dissected aorta.

### Protocol

MRI is safe to use with almost all mechanical valve replacements although local guidelines should be followed.[1]

Standard safety checks should be performed.

- ECG-gated imaging.
- Localizers followed by ultrafast axial images for planning.
- Sagittal oblique dark blood images to assess the aortic dimensions.
- Phase contrast flow images at the level of the aortic valve looking for regurgitation.
- Contrast enhanced aortic MR angiography.

### Angiography

Catheter angiography for the diagnosis and follow-up of aortic aneurysms has been largely superseded by non-invasive techniques such as CT and MRI. Angiography may be required to assess the coronary arteries prior to surgery.

## Differential diagnosis

CT, MRI, echocardiography and angiography are sensitive and specific for thoracic aortic aneurysm.

## Management

Treatment depends on the aetiology, size and complications of the aneurysm.

- Aneurysms may be followed-up by serial imaging if small and uncomplicated.
- Surgical repair carries a significant morbidity and mortality depending on the location and complications.
- Endovascular stenting of the thoracic aorta is a rapidly developing field. It is predominantly used for descending aortic disease. Fenestrated stents and ascending aortic devices are in development.

## Complications
- See also clinical features above
- Aortic regurgitation from dilatation of the aortic root
- Sinus of Valsalva aneurysms
- Rupture

## Further reading

**1.** Further information can also be found at http://www.mrisafety.com.

**2.** Yu T, Zhu X, Tang L et al. (2007) Review of CT angiography of aorta. *Radiol Clin N Am* **45**; 461–83.

**3.** Sakamoto I, Sueyoshi E and Uetani M (2007) MR imaging of the aorta. *Radiol Clin N Am* **45**; 485–97.

**4.** Johnson TR et al. (2007) ECG-gated 64-MDCT angiography in the differential diagnosis of acute chest pain. *AJR* 2007; **188**; 76–82.

# Myocardial infarction and acute coronary syndrome

Myocardial infarction (MI) is necrosis of cardiac muscle tissue caused by ischaemia. Acute coronary syndrome (ACS) is an umbrella term for several clinical manifestations of coronary artery disease including unstable angina, ST-elevation MI (STEMI) and non-ST-elevation MI (NSTEMI).

## Aetiology and epidemiology

MI is usually secondary to the acute rupture of a coronary artery atherosclerotic plaque with subsequent thrombosis leading to occlusion of the vessel and thus diminished blood supply to the heart muscle. ACS is usually due to a lesser form of stenosis or occlusion.

## Clinical features and non-imaging investigations

Clinical features of both MI and ACS include acute crushing central chest pain with radiation into the neck and left arm, sweating, nausea and vomiting and cardiovascular collapse. Heart failure and dysrhythmias are also common.

The initial diagnosis is usually made on history, physical examination, ECG and elevated cardiac serum enzymes (preferably Troponin I but also Troponin T and CK-MB; the troponins are more sensitive and specific then CK-MB). Timing of the blood tests is important and should be taken 6–9hrs after the time of insult.

## Imaging

The role of imaging in the setting of ACS is limited if the diagnosis is clear. Imaging is reserved for clarifying diagnosis in difficult cases and/or for assessment of complications. Aortic dissection and pulmonary embolus are the main differential diagnoses that imaging can exclude. Contrast-enhanced MRI can be used to assess the acute and chronic changes to the heart following myocardial infarction.

The use of CXR, echo, cardiac CT and cardiac MRI may all add additional information regarding the diagnosis; however, the importance of rapid medical, catheter-based or surgical treatment may preclude their use in the acute setting.

Cardiac CT in particular is finding an emerging role in the evaluation of acute chest pain presenting to the emergency department.

The major benefit of cardiac CT in the emergency situation is its high negative predictive value: a normal CT has a >98% NPV for coronary disease.

## Cardiac CT

### Protocol

- Unenhanced examination to measure the calcium score
- ECG-gated, contrast-enhanced imaging for the coronary arteries.
- Reconstruction of data at multiple points during the cardiac cycle to assess each of the major coronary vessels
- The use of MIPs, MPRs and VRTs is essential to fully evaluate the heart. The remainder of the chest must be reviewed to look for any lung/chest wall abnormality.

The role of the 'Triple Rule Out' scan to assess coronary artery disease, pulmonary emboli and aortic dissection is gaining popularity. It is technically feasible to image the entire chest with ECG-gating in one breath-hold with high quality images of the pulmonary, systemic and cardiac vessels (📖 p. 61).

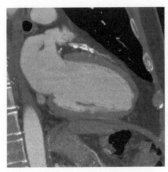

**Fig. 6.4** Oblique MPR from a cardiac CT demonstrating calcification in the left coronary artery.

### Differential diagnosis

- Aortic dissection
- Pulmonary embolus
- Causes of an acute abdomen
- Myocarditis
- Pericarditis

Acute myocardial infarction is not the only cause of an elevated serum troponin level. Other differentials must be considered, especially if there is some doubt in diagnosis, e.g. acute PE, acute pericarditis, acute or severe heart failure, myocarditis, sepsis, shock, renal failure, false-positive elevated troponin.

### Management

The management of acute myocardial infarction is directed towards re-establishing a blood supply to the ischaemic myocardium to prevent further cell death and thus preserve myocardial function. Treatments include thrombolysis (e.g. streptokinase, rtPA), anti-platelet therapy (e.g. aspirin), beta-blockers, nitrates and heparin.

Primary percutaneous coronary intervention (PCI) with either angioplasty or stenting is becoming increasingly common in selected cases.

The majority of the management of acute myocardial infarction in the UK is undertaken by the cardiology team with little radiological input although there are regional variations depending on experience. Radiology plays a greater role in chronic management or where there is diagnostic uncertainty; in particular cardiac MRI (for ischaemia burden and viability imaging) and cardiac CT (coronary anatomy and other causes of chest pain) play an important role.

## Complications

- Dysrhythmias, both ventricular and supra-ventricular
- Conduction abnormalities
- Heart failure
- Myocardial rupture/ischaemic VSD
- Ischaemic mitral regurgitation
- LV aneurysm formation
- Cardiogenic shock

**Further reading**

**1.** Roongsritong C et al. (2004) common causes of troponin elevations in the absence of acute myocardial infarction: incidence and clinical significance *Chest* **125**; 1877–84.

**2.** White CS and Kuo D (2007) Chest pain in the emergency department: role of multidetector CT. *Radiology* **245**; 672–81.

**3.** Schopef UJ, Zwerner PL, Savino G et al. (2007) Coronary CT angiography. *Radiology* **244**; 48–63.

**4.** Jaffe AS, Rvkilde J, Roberts R et al. (2000) It's time for a change to a troponin standard. *Circulation* **102**; 1216–20.

# :✪: **Abdominal aortic aneurysm (AAA)**

Pathological dilatation of the abdominal aorta by over 50% of its normal diameter (>3cm although there is no clear consensus).

## Aetiology/risk factors

- Commonest in white males >75 years old.
- Prior atherosclerotic vascular disease.
- Smoking.
- Hypertension.
- Positive family history.

## Clinical features

- Aneurysm intact:
  - Asymptomatic
  - Abdominal mass
  - Abdominal pain
- Leaking/ruptured:
  - Sudden onset of abdominal pain
  - Distended abdomen
  - Hypotension
  - Circulatory collapse

## Imaging

In the setting of a leaking/ruptured AAA, the haemodynamically unstable patient should be taken immediately to theatre at the discretion of the vascular surgeon. The stable patient should be assessed with CT, in particular to assess suitability for endovascular repair.

### Radiographs

Plain abdominal radiography plays no part in the management of a patient suspected of have a leaking AAA as it only delays definitive imaging/treatment and has a low sensitivity.

*Findings*

- May be normal or show mural calcification
- Loss of the psoas shadow may represent retroperitoneal bleeding

### US

FAST (Focused Assessment with Sonography in Trauma) has become a widespread US technique employed in the emergency department by emergency physicians which is used to rapidly detect the presence of free fluid within the abdominal cavity (🕮 p. 69). The technique is poor for assessment of retroperitoneal fluid and was developed primarily for use in haemodynamically unstable patients after blunt abdominal trauma. Whilst FAST can be rapidly performed in the resuscitation scenario, it lacks both sensitivity and specificity, especially in inexperienced hands.

*Findings*

Highly accurate at assessing aneurysm size.

### CT

CT examination should be performed only if the patient is haemodynamically stable.

*Protocol*

The CT examination of AAA is similar for thoracic dissection (📖 p. 115). Bolus triggering is the fastest way of achieving arterial phase imaging.

- NECT: this is used to size the aneurysm. It may be all that is required to prove the presence of haematoma around the aneurysm and thus indicate a leak that requires surgical management.
- There is an argument for not performing a CECT following the NECT if the diagnosis of leak or rupture is evident, thus sparing a dose of nephrotoxic contrast medium. If endovascular aneurysm repair (EVAR) is being considered then a CECT is mandatory to allow planning.

*Findings*

- A mass or collection in the perirenal space may be seen. The aorta may be displaced anteriorly. Mixed attenuation 'soft tissue' mass around the aorta is the haematoma.
- Extravasation of contrast medium may be seen in acute rupture.
- Sizing the aneurysm is important. Arterial images should be obtained from the aortic hiatus and should include the femoral vessels. This wide coverage will define the neck, the relation to the renal arteries and the tortuosity of the iliac vessels, thus allowing planning for endovascular repair or open surgery as appropriate. The majority of aneurysms are infra-renal, however for safe endovascular repair, a neck of at least 1cm is required.
- If the aorta is dilated at the hiatus then consideration should be given to imaging the thoracic aorta in addition.
- Multiplanar reconstructions are mandatory for assessing anatomical relations.
- If the CT study is negative then features of renal calculi and pancreatitis should be sought as these may mimic the presentation of AAA. Acute myocardial infarction/acute coronary syndrome should also be considered.

## MRI

MRI is excellent for assessing aneurysm size although it plays no part in the management of an acute rupture or leak.

## Management

With acute leak or rupture, urgent surgical or endovascular repair are the only potentially life-saving interventions.

## Complications of treatment

- Death: 1.8–5% if elective and 50% if ruptured.
- Renal failure.
- Myocardial infarction: 2–5%.
- Graft infection (rare).
- Colon ischaemia (more common if ruptured).

## Further reading

**1.** Macura KJ, Corl FM, Fishman EK *et al.* (2003) Pathogenesis in acute aortic syndromes: aortic aneurysm leak and rupture and traumatic aortic transection. *Am J Roentgen* **181**; 303–7.

**2.** Salvolini L, Reanda P, Fiore D *et al.* (2008) Acute aortic syndromes: role of multidetector row CT. *Eur J Radiol* **65**(3); 350–8.

# Traumatic great vessel injury

The majority of great vessel injuries are caused by rapid deceleration, especially as a result of an RTA.

Other causes include:
- falls from a significant height
- blast injuries
- collisions between pedestrians and vehicles

## Clinical features

The patient may present in variety of ways. Acute chest pain following trauma, hypotension and shock, suspicion on CXR or as an incidental finding due to investigation for polytrauma are common presentations.

## Imaging

Patients presenting with a history of deceleration injury, major chest wall injury, fractures to the 1st or 2nd ribs or sternoclavicular joint dislocation should be considered at high risk for traumatic great vessel injury.

Associated injury to the head and neck vessels is uncommon although it should be considered when suspicion of aortic injury is present.

Superior vena cava (SVC) and inferior vena cava (IVC) injury are unusual from blunt trauma. IVC and SVC injury should be suspected if a traumatic pericardial effusion is present. Damage to the intrapericardial IVC should be carefully excluded in any major hepatic injury.

### CXR

*Protocol*

Often the presenting film is a supine portable radiograph taken in the emergency department as part of the 3-film trauma series (CXR, lateral cervical spine and AP pelvis).

*Findings*
- The CXR is unreliable for excluding great vessel injury, especially when only a suboptimal emergency film is available.
- A number of signs that suggest mediastinal haematoma, and therefore great vessel injury, have been described and these include:
  - Widening of the mediastinum
  - Obscuration of the aortic knuckle or distortion of the aortic contour
  - Right paratracheal soft tissue mass
  - Displacement of the oesophagus to the right
  - All can be the result of a false positive due to pleural effusion, atelectasis, motion, lines and tubes or mediastinal fat
- Major chest wall injury seen on CXR should raise the suspicion of great vessel inury.

### CT

This is the imaging modality of choice if great vessel injury is suspected and has now largely superseded catheter angiography as the 'gold standard'.

*Protocol*
- Oral contrast medium not required.
- Unenhanced images through the chest and upper abdomen to assess for haematoma.

- Arterial phase images starting in the neck, extending to the aortic bifurcation; either bolus triggered or with test-bolus timing.
- Consider portal and delayed phase imaging of the abdomen and pelvis.
- All images should be reviewed with multiplanar reformats (MPRs).

*Findings*
- NECT: The purpose of the unenhanced imaging is to look for high density (60–80HU), fresh haematoma within the vessel wall suggesting trauma to the vessel. Lung injury, pneumothorax, haemothorax and fractures can also be assessed with these images.
- CECT (arterial): In the arterial phase the mediastinal contents will be fully delineated. Common signs include:
  - Pseudoaneurysm (dilatation of an artery with disruption of one or more layers of its walls, rather than with expansion of all wall layers)
  - Periaortic haematoma
  - Displacement of mediastinal structures away from the aorta
  - Intimal flaps projecting into the vessel lumen
  - Luminal clot at the site of intimal tears
  - Calibre changes within the aorta
  - Transection of the aorta (rare)
  - Active extravasation of contrast medium from the aorta into the pleural cavity or mediastinum
- It is of the utmost importance that the whole of the aorta and great vessels be analysed fully as injury can occur anywhere along the length of the aorta. The commonest location for injury is just distal to the origin of the left brachiocephalic trunk.
- To aid the interventional radiologist or surgeon, the following should be noted:
  - The precise location of the injury/injuries
  - Length of injury
  - Relationship of the injured segment to major aortic branches and if the branch vessels are involved
  - Any intraluminal thrombus
  - The size of the aorta both proximal and distal to the lesion(s)
  - The presence of any congenital anomalies related to the aorta or its branches

*Angiography*
The ease and availability of CT, its non-invasive nature, and the facility to fully evaluate the polytrauma patient have changed the role of angiography. Catheter angiography should be used where diagnostic doubt is still present after CT or for therapeutic intervention with stents.

## Management

- As a traumatic injury to the aorta or the great vessels is a potentially fatal injury, urgent treatment is required once the diagnosis has been made.
- Endoluminal stenting of even complex injuries is possible.
- Urgent cardiothoracic surgical intervention may be required.

## Further reading

**1.** Mirvis SE (2006) Thoracic vascular injury. *Radiol Clin N Am* **44**; 181–97.

# Traumatic peripheral arterial and venous injury

For the purposes of this chapter, arterial and venous injury will be considered together.

## Aetiology

- Penetrating injury: violence, industrial, iatrogenic
- Blunt trauma: RTAs, falls, crush/blast injuries
- Fractured long bones, supracondylar fractures of the humerus and femur
- Dislocations: elbow, posterior knee, shoulder

## Clinical features

Symptoms and signs of distal ischaemia include pain, pallor, paralysis, parasthesa, pulselessness, prolonged capillary refill (the 6 'P's).

Other signs include: observed bleeding which is pulsatile if arterial; arterial thrill/bruit; visibly expanding haematoma.

## Imaging

### Radiographs

This has no direct role in imaging the vascular injury but may be used to exclude or assess for associated fractures, dislocations and foreign bodies.

### Angiography

May be performed either in the catheter laboratory ('cath lab') or in the operating theatre and can fully delineate both arterial and venous injury Angiography is the main imaging modality for such abnormalities.

- Standard vascular access techniques.

### CT

CT is often performed as a first line investigation in the polytrauma patient. Whilst CT is not the ideal imaging modality for assessing peripheral vascular injury, it can be used to examine the larger vessels, in particular arteries.

#### Protocol

Standard trauma protocols should be used. It is important with modern CT scanners that the contrast bolus is not 'out-run' (i.e. the imaging is performed before the contrast reaches the vessel of interest) by either having too short a delay or too high a pitch, especially for imaging the legs. Precise timings for arterial imaging should be adjusted depending on coverage required. For venous imaging delayed images should be acquired 60–120s after contrast medium injection.

*Findings*

- In patients with polytrauma, contrast-enhanced CT may demonstrate the affects of vascular injury. Discontinuities in the column of contrast in vessels, extravasation of contrast medium and haematoma can be assessed particularly in the arterial system.
- The study should be carefully reviewed to assess peripheral vessels. The use of MPRs and MIP reconstruction is very useful.

## Management

- Following minor injury, conservative management can be adopted with repeated clinical examination to assess for deterioration. Investigations such as ultrasound can be performed serially. Angiography and CT are usually required for more major injury or when significant deterioration in the patient's condition has occurred.
- In major injury, surgical management is usually appropriate.
- Angiographic stenting may be useful for localized lesions.

## Complications

- Nerve damage
- Compartment syndrome
- Venous thrombosis
- Arterial embolisation
- Limb loss

## Further reading

**1.** McGahan JP, Richards J and Fogata ML (2004) Emergency ultrasound in trauma patients. *Radiol Clin N Am* **42**; 417–25.

**2.** Miller-Thomas MM, Clark West O and Cohen AM (2005) Diagnosing traumatic arterial injury in the extremities with CT angiography: perils and pitfalls. *Radiographics* **25**(Suppl. 1); S133–42.

# ⑦ Deep vein thrombosis

The presence of thrombus in one of the deep venous channels. It can become fragmented and result in a potentially fatal pulmonary embolus.

## Aetiology and epidemiology

The pathophysiology relates to the Virchow triad of venous stasis, vessel wall injury and a hypercoagulable state. Risk factors include immobility, recent surgery, malignancy, obesity and previous DVT.

Lower limb DVT is the commonest site with a population prevalence of 1 in 1000.

## Clinical features and non-imaging investigations

- Can be asymptomatic.
- Often non-specific symptoms, e.g. pain and swelling of the affected limb.
- The D-dimer is a fibrin degradation product and its serum level is elevated in venous thrombotic disease. It is also raised in other conditions, e.g. pregnancy, malignancy and post-surgery. Since these conditions themselves predispose to DVT formation they make the D-dimer assay unreliable in such cases. However, a normal D-dimer has a strong negative predictive value.

## Imaging

DVT imaging does not need to be performed as an emergency unless there is a contraindication to anticoagulation. The majority of patients can be started on therapeutic dose low molecular weight heparin (LMWH) and imaged the next day.

In the presence of PE, imaging for DVT is not usually indicated. Although the presence of a DVT can add weight to the diagnosis of PE, the presence of normal leg veins does not exclude PE as a likely diagnosis.

### US

US has a very high negative predictive value (99.5%[1]).

*Protocol*
- 5–10Mhz linear transducer
- Imaging from groin (proximal common femoral vein) to popliteal fossa is sufficient to exclude a significant DVT. Some centres advocate that imaging at the popliteal fossa and groin only (without imaging of the vessels in between) is sufficient to exclude a significant DVT.
- Compress the vein in the AP direction until there is apposition of the walls indicating a patent vein. The pressure required to do this is always less than would be required to compress the accompanying artery.
- Colour Doppler examination provides a more comprehensive examination: colour should fill the vessel lumen with no aliasing outside the vessels. Aliasing occurs when the Doppler gain is set too high and random colour is seen outside the vessel wall in the surrounding soft tissue. It is important that the gate gain settings be adjusted to maintain sensitivity whilst reducing artefact.
- The flow pattern in the vessel can be interrogated by pulse wave Doppler during: augmentation of flow by squeezing of the calf; during respiratory variation by asking the patient to breathe deeply; or during

the Valsalva manoeuvre (forcibly exhaling against a closed glottis). If the vessel is patent, flow should vary during all three manoeuvres. When diagnosis is unclear, then imaging of the contra-lateral leg using the same manoeuvres is of benefit.

*Findings*
- Acute thrombus may be anechoic, therefore lack of compressibility and a filling defect on colour imaging is needed to confirm DVT.
- Clot may be visualized as a hyperechoic mass.
- Failure to fully compress indicates occlusion of the vessel.
- Once the presence of DVT has been established it is important to define the proximal extent by imaging the iliac veins as far as possible.

Normal appearances transverse grayscale US

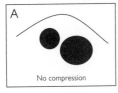

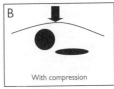

DVT: Longitudinal Doppler US

DVT: Transverse grayscale US

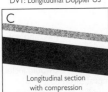

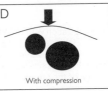

**Fig. 6.5** Schematic US appearances of the right common femoral vessels on grayscale US (A, B, D) and Doppler US (C). Both the normal appearances (A, B) and the appearances with a DVT (C, D) are shown. The vein is normally larger and fully compressible compared to the artery. On Doppler US in the presence of a DVT, the artery fills with colour flow whereas there is no flow in the expanded thrombosed vein.

*Other modalities*

CT and MRI are of limited use in the routine detection of DVT, although both have a high sensitivity and specificity. These techniques are of use in difficult cases. DVT can also be an incidental finding during abdominal and pelvic CT/MRI. All such studies should be carefully evaluated to exclude incidental DVT. Some centres have advocated delayed imaging (90–120s) of the pelvic veins following a PE study. The presence of a DVT with a negative PE study will ensure that anticoagulation is commenced. However, the dose to the pelvis, especially in women of child-bearing age, should be considered.

- When US is negative, some centres will repeat this within 7 days to exclude a below-knee DVT that has propagated above the knee.
- Other methods such as MR venography and venogram could be considered in difficult cases or when there is suspicion of thrombus in the pelvic vessels.

### Differential diagnosis

- Muscle trauma
- Ruptured Baker's cyst
- Thrombophlebitis
- Cellulitis
- Arterial insufficiency
- Lymphoedema

### Management

- Initial anticoagulation with LMWH or heparin and thromboembolic deterrent (TED) stockings. Full anticoagulation with warfarin for 3–6 months with an International Normalized Ratio (INR) = 2.
- IVC filter if there is a significant risk of PE. Such risk would include recurrent PE or the presence of iliofemoral thrombus.

### Complications

- Related to the thrombus:
  - Clot extension to more proximal vessels including the IVC
  - Clot fragmentation leading to PE
  - Venous insufficiency following damage to the deep venous system with long term consequences including varicose veins
- Related to anticoagulation:
  - Bleeding

### Further reading

**1.** Subramaniam RM, Heath R, Chou T et al. (2005) Deep venous thrombosis: withholding anticoagulation therapy after negative complete lower limb US findings. *Radiology* **237**; 348–52.

**2.** Scarsbrook AF, Evans AL, Owen AR et al. (2006) Diagnosis of suspected venous thromboembolic disease in pregnancy. *Clin Rad* **61**; 1–12.

**3.** Rumack CM, Wilson SR, Charboneau JW and Johnson J-A (2004) *Diagnostic Ultrasound*, 3rd edn, Mosby.

# Central venous catheter assessment

The assessment of central venous catheters (CVCs) is important both at the time of insertion and if complications are suspected.

200 000 CVCs are inserted in the UK per year and are used for: haemodynamic monitoring, fluid replacement, haemodialysis, total parenteral nutrition (TPN) and delivery of blood products and drugs.

## Classification

CVCs may be classified into four groups:
- peripherally inserted central catheters (PICCs)
- temporary (non-tunnelled) CVCs
- permanent (tunnelled) CVCs
- implantable ports

PICC lines are placed in the antecubital fossa and generally used for short to intermediate term administration of drugs or TPN. Tunnelled lines such as Hickman lines and Vascaths (for heamofiltration/dialysis) are inserted into a central vein then tunnelled to emerge on the chest wall some distance from the vein. This is to prevent infection. Such lines can be used in the longer term. Implantable ports are similar to tunnelled lines except that they are completely buried in the subcutaneous tissue. These are accessed using specifically designed needles and are best used for intermittent administration of drugs such as antibiotics e.g. in the cystic fibrosis population.

## Imaging

### Radiographs

*Protocol*

The CXR is the main form of imaging used to assess a CVC. Usually a film is taken soon after the insertion of the line to assess both its position and any immediate complications such as pneumothorax or haemothorax (📖 p. 90). Inspiratory and expiratory films may be helpful in detecting a small pneumothorax. The ideal form of imaging is a departmental PA (posteroanterior) CXR but often only a portable CXR of reduced quality can be obtained in practice.

*Findings*

- The precise position of the tip of the line and how to assess it are controversial.
- **Single lumen lines**: the tip should lie within the SVC as can be judged by the carina: the tip should lie at the level of the carina.
- **Double lumen lines** used for haemodialysis: the tip should be within the right atrium.
- Change in posture can affect the position of a line. Serial films may be useful to assess migration of the tip or evolving complications.

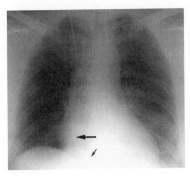

**Fig. 6.6** CXR demonstrating a CVC (large arrow) that has been inserted too far: the tip (small arrow) can be seen within the heart.

### Fluoroscopy

Fluoroscopy is often used to check line patency, tip position and to assess leakage around the line insertion site which can be due to fracture of the line.

*Protocol and findings*

- The patient should be consented, either verbally or in writing, and is usually positioned supine.
- After control images have been taken, the skin and CVC should be cleaned and treated using aseptic technique.
- Each port on the line should be flushed in turn with IV contrast medium (e.g. Iopamidol 300) while continuously screening. It should be injected slowly and no force should be necessary to flush the line. The contrast medium should fill the line and flow freely away towards the heart. If contrast does not flow freely some form of obstruction should be assumed and no further force used.
- The insertion site should be observed to assess for leaking onto the skin surface. Any extravasation of contrast is abnormal.
- Once all ports have been checked the line(s) should be flushed with either saline or heparinised saline as appropriate.

### Ultrasound

Ultrasound guidance is increasingly being used to aid CVC insertion and to lessen complication rates.

Ultrasound can also be used to assess the central veins of the head and neck and groin prior to CVC insertion or when complications such as central venous thrombosis or vessel stenosis are suspected. This can occur if multiple CVCs have been used or in sick patients with a pro-thrombotic state.

Thrombosed vessels show echo bright thrombus in the lumen, decreased or absent flow and are non-compressible. Stenosis may be demonstrated by the visualization of discrete narrowing, flow acceleration through the stenosis or altered haemodynamics with respiration (📖 p. 132 DVT).

*Other modalities*

CT, MRI and angiography have no part to play in the first line assessment of CVC complications or position; this is the remit of the CXR. All three modalities do however play an important role in the assessment of:

• abnormalities found on the initial CXR
• longer term complications such as venous stenosis or occlusion
• the location of the distal segment if the line fractures

Standard protocols are beyond the scope of this text.

## Differential diagnosis of CVC complications

### Immediate

Failure to cannulate vein, arterial puncture, bleeding, dysrhythmias, air embolus.

### Early

Haematoma, pneumothorax, haemothorax, pneumomediastinum.

Early complications occur either immediately or become apparent within few hours of the line being inserted.

### Late

Infection (at the insertion site as well as distant from it), thrombosis, extravasation, SVC obstruction.

Late complications can occur days to months after lines have been inserted, especially when the line has been left *in situ* for an extended period of time, or lines have been repeatedly inserted into the same vessel.

SVC obstruction (SVCO) is most commonly secondary to malignancy although the commonest benign cause is the use of intravascular devices. Facial, neck and upper extremity swelling, dyspnoea at rest, cough and dilated chest wall veins are the usual mode of presentation.

## Further reading

**1.** Poldeman KH and Girbes AR (2002) Central venous catheter use. Part 1: mechanical complications and Part 2: infectious complications. *Intensive Care Medicine* **28**; 1–28.

**2.** McGee DC and Gould MK (2003) Preventing complications of central venous catherization. *New England Journal of Medicine* **348**; 1123–33.

**3.** Arnchick JM and Miller WT Jr (1997) Tubes and lines in the intensive care setting. *Seminars in Roentgenology* **33**; 102–16.

**4.** Maecken TD and Grau T (2007) Ultrasound imaging in vascular access. *Critical Care Medicine* **35**(Suppl.); S178–85.

**5.** Tan PL and Gibson M (2007) Central venous catheters: the role of radiology. *Clinical Radiology* **61**; 13–22.

**6.** Burney K, Young H, Barnard SA et al. (2007) CT appearances of congenital and acquired abnormalities of the superior vena cava. *Clinical Radiology* **62**; 837–42.

## Pericardial effusion

# ① ⑦ **Pericardial effusion**

An abnormal collection of fluid in the pericardial space: 15–20ml of fluid may be seen on CT.

## Aetiology and epidemiology

A wide range of etiologies can cause a pericardial effusion. These include malignancy (primary pericardial and secondary deposits), myocardial infarction, infection (viral, pyogenic, tuberculous and fungal), uraemia, heart failure, aortic dissection, and autoimmune diseases.

Malignant effusions are the commonest cause as a result of secondary deposits, although the presence of a pericardial effusion in the context of malignancy does not imply invasion of the pericardium. Lung, breast and lymphoma are the commonest malignant causes.

## Clinical features and non-imaging investigations

### Clinical

- Beck's triad: increased JVP, hypotension, diminished heart sounds.
- Pulsus paradoxus: an exaggeration of the normal inspiratory decrease in systolic BP (>12 mmHg).
- Kussmaul respiration: usually seen in constrictive pericarditis; paradoxical increase in venous distension during inspiration.

### ECG

The following 12-lead ECG changes are suggestive of, but not diagnostic for, a pericardial effusion: sinus tachycardia, low-voltage QRS complexes PR segment depression.

## Imaging

### Radiographs

Plain radiography of the chest can be normal even with a small but haemodynamically significant effusion. An enlarged cardiac silhouette with a globular configuration is the classic CXR appearance.

### Chest ultrasound/echocardiography

Pericardial effusions may be seen incidentally when imaging the chest. They appear as an anechoic/hypoechoic layer surrounding the heart, bounded by the pericardium. In cases of haematoma or infection the collection may have a more complex echogenicity appearance.

Echocardiography is usually performed by cardiologists and is a quick bedside investigation that allows both diagnosis and treatment with pericardiocentesis if appropriate.

### CT

#### Protocol

Non-contrast enhanced imaging through the pericardial sac followed by an arterial phase volume acquisition through the chest. Delayed imaging at 60s can be performed to assess pericardial enhancement. CT parameters as the same as for any other CT of the chest.

*Findings*
- CECT easily detects ~20ml of pericardial fluid. Small effusions can be frequently missed on thoracic NECT or on abdominal CT when the views of the pericardial space are limited.
- CT can also indicate the presence of cardiac tamponade: this is suggested if the ventricles, especially the right, are compressed and the atria dilated. This is also seen with constrictive pericarditis.
- CECT may also give an indication of the etiology of the effusion. The presence of loculated fluid and pericardial thickening (>2mm) should be noted: these are more likely if the cause is infective. The Hounsfield unit value of the pericardial fluid may also give an indication as to etiology: a density similar to water suggests a simple effusion whereas high density fluid suggests blood, fluid due to malignancy, or pus. Furthermore, imaging of the rest of the chest and upper abdomen may demonstrate an underlying malignancy.

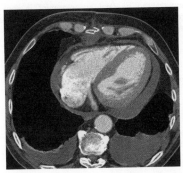

**Fig. 6.7** Pericardial effusion demonstrated on an axial CT image. Note also the bilateral pleural effusions.

### Pericardiocentesis and US/CT guided drainage
Pericardiocentesis can be performed without radiological guidance (see ref. 2) but US (echo)-guidance is preferential to avoid complications. Pericardial drainage is usually performed under US (echo)-guidance. However, a pericardial collection can also be aspirated or drained safely with CT guidance when the size or location of the fluid makes US (echo)-guided techniques difficult or impossible (see 📖 p. 378 for aspiration and drain insertion).

### Protocol
The pericardial space can be entered from either side using a parasternal approach or more laterally from a left anterior approach. Ideally the pleural space should not be entered. Standard Seldinger techniques are used and dedicated pericardial drains (Van Sonnenberg) or pigtail drains up to 10 Fr can be inserted.

### Differential diagnosis

- Acute myocardial infarction
- Pericarditis
- Cardiac tamponade

Once the presence of pericardial fluid has been established the cause should be elucidated.

## Management

Effusions not causing haemodynamic compromise may be treated conservatively with treatment of the underlying cause.

When cardiac tamponade is present, or even suspected, then US (echo)-guided pericardiocentesis is the procedure of choice. Other treatment options available include CT-guided aspiration/drainage or the formation of a pericardial window which is a surgical procedure.

## Complications

Cardiac tamponade can be fatal so treatment is required urgently. Pericardiocentesis may be complicated by damage to the epicardial vessels or myocardium, pneumothorax, infection or dysryhthmia.

**Further reading**

**1.** Wang ZH, Reddy GP, Gotway MB *et al.* (2003) CT and MR imaging of pericardial disease. *RadioGraphics* **23**; S167–80.

**2.** Longmore M, Wilkinson IB, Turmezei T, Cheung CH, (2008) *Oxford Handbook of Clinical Medicine*, 7e, Oxford: Oxford University Press; 761.

# Gastrointestinal

# ⦸ Acute appendicitis

### Aetiology and epidemiology

Inflammation of the appendix is usually secondary to obstruction of the appendicular orifice which, if untreated, proceeds to perforation of the appendix. It is the most common cause of acute abdominal pain requiring surgery. It is most common in the second decade of life, but can occur at any age.

### Clinical features

Migratory right iliac fossa pain, fever, vomiting, diarrhoea, rebound tenderness at McBurney's point.

### Imaging

Does suspected appendicitis require imaging, and if so which modality should be used? There is no consensus on this issue, except that US should be performed first on premenopausal women to exclude gynaecological pathology.

US is poor at excluding appendicitis when the appendix is not visualized. Although high rates of visualization of the appendix are quoted in the literature (86%[1]), many find it difficult to replicate these results. If visualized, the sensitivity for appendicitis is high (98%[1]). US can be useful to exclude abscess formation in patients in whom laparoscopic resection is being considered.

CT has a high sensitivity and specificity (both 98% in one study[2]), but radiation dose limits its use in young people, and it should be used sparingly in children. Many centres employ a clinical scoring system, the Alvarado score.[3] Patients with a high score are scheduled for surgery, those with a low score are observed or discharged and only those with an intermediate score are examined by CT.

### *Ultrasound*

*Protocol*

Abdominal and pelvic ultrasound (full urinary bladder advised) using 3–6MHz curvilinear probe. Consider endovaginal examination in appropriate circumstances (sexually mature women, appropriate experience and chaperones available). Examination of the appendix is by graded compression over the right iliac fossa using a linear probe (6–15MHz). The appendix is identified as a blind-ending tubular structure attached to the posteromedial border of the caecal pole. The caecum is usually visualized as a gas-filled structure in the right iliac fossa. The terminal ileum may be mistaken for the appendix, but has an attachment to the medial wall of the colon and is not blind-ending.

*Findings*

An inflamed appendix is identified as follows:
• Incompressible
• Has an external diameter >6mm (when pressure is applied)
• May demonstrate an appendicolith (very echogenic mass with acoustic shadow)
• Aperistaltic
• Painful to compression
• Increased blood flow within the wall on Doppler interrogation

If the appendix is not identified, inflammation of the pericaecal fat (demonstrated as reduced echogenicity) and free fluid in the right iliac fossa are features suggestive of appendicitis.

If appendicitis is diagnosed, look for generalized free peritoneal fluid or abscess formation indicating perforation.

## CT

*Protocol*
- 2.5–5mm reconstructions
- Oral contrast to fill caecum: preferably 40min to 1h prior to examination.
- 100–150ml IV contrast injected at 3–4ml/s, with image acquisition at 60s.

Dedicated examination of only the right iliac fossa after a large volume of rectal contrast (but without oral or IV contrast) has been advocated but is not generally accepted.[2]

*Findings*
- Identify appendix: blind ending tube arising from the tip of the caecum.
- The 6mm diameter used as the upper limit of normal for compression US does not apply to CT, as the appendix is not compressed. 10mm should be used instead.[4]
- A thick wall that is hyperenhancing favours appendicitis, although a necrotic appendix will have failure of enhancement.
- Appendicolith is a calcified mass within the appendix lumen. Often this has a laminated appearance. This can be found in 7% of normal patients.[4] If the appendix has perforated, the appendicolith may be seen within an abscess cavity.
- Inflammatory changes in periappendicular fat with fluid collections.
- 'Arrowhead' sign: inflammatory changes around the appendix orifice produce a cone shape that fills with oral contrast.
- Failure of oral contrast to enter the appendix (historically failure of barium to enter the appendix during a barium enema was used as a sign of acute appendicitis). Distal appendicitis may occur, however, with a normal proximal appendix that fills with contrast.
- Look for complications:
  - Perforation: abdominal/pelvic free fluid
  - Abscess formation
  - Small bowel obstruction (📖 p. 152)

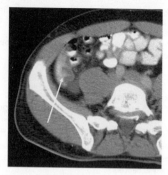

**Fig.7.1** Abdominal CT showing arrowhead sign in caecum (arrow).

## Differential diagnoses

- Terminal ileitis of Crohn's disease
- Ovarian cyst (📖 p. 306)
- Ovarian torsion (📖 p. 310)
- Mesenteric adenitis
- Right sided diverticulitis (📖 p. 148)
- Renal/ureteric colic (📖 p. 192)
- Ectopic pregnancy (📖 p. 322)
- Typhlitis (infectious inflammation of the caecum in immunocompromised patients)
- Caecal tumour
- Epiploic appendagitis (see Diverticulitis 📖 p. 148)

## Further reading

**1.** Kessler N, Cyteval C, Gallix B et al. (2004) Appendicitis: evaluation of sensitivity, specificity, and predictive values of US, Doppler US, and laboratory fingings. *Radiology* **230**; 472–8.

**2.** Rao PM, Rhea Jt, Novelline RA et al. (1997) Helical CT combined with contrast material administered only through the colon for imaging of suspected appendicitis. *AJR* **169**; 1275–80.

**3.** Douglas CD, Macpherson NE, Davidson PM et al. (2000) Randomised controlled trial of ultrasonography in diagnosis of acute appendicitis, incorporating the Alvarado score. *BMJ* **321**(7266); 919–22.

**4.** Benjaminov O, Atri M, Hamilton P et al. (2002) Frequency of visualization and thickness of normal appendix at non-enhanced helical CT. *Radiology* **225**; 400–6.

**5.** Rao PM, Rhea JT, Rattner DW et al. (1999) Introduction of appendiceal CT: impact on negative appendectomy and appendiceal perforation rates. *Ann Surg* **229**(3); 344–9.

# ⊙ Diverticulitis

## Epidemiology

Diverticulosis is a common condition in Western countries, and incidence increases with increasing age: 50% over 50 years of age. Inflammation (diverticulitis) occurs in 10–25% people with diverticulitis. Perforation and abscess formation may complicate, and in the long term, strictures. Fistulation into the bladder is relatively common in the elderly; look for gas in a bladder that has not been recently catheterized.

Right-sided diverticulitis tends to be limited in extent, sometimes to a single diverticulum, and runs a more benign course.

## Clinical features

Lower abdominal pain, fever, diarrhoea, signs of sepsis.

## Imaging

### CT

CT is generally the first-line investigation.

*Protocol*
- Coverage from diaphragm to pubic symphysis
- Oral contrast medium 20min prior to study
- 5mm reconstructions or thinner
- 100–150ml IV contrast at 3–4ml/s, with image acquisition at 60s

*Findings*
- Ill-defined high attenuation in the fat around the inflamed segment of bowel. Bowel wall thickening is often associated. Look for free gas in the peritoneum, in the sigmoid mesocolon, and retroperitoneum.
- Stricture identified by dilatation of proximal large bowel, with liquid contents.
- An abscess is demonstrated as a fluid attenuation mass ± gas, with a thick, enhancing wall adjacent to an inflamed area of bowel.

### Ultrasound

*Protocol*
3–6MHz curvilinear probe.

*Findings*
The usefulness of US is limited due to bowel gas. Rings of hypoechoic, inflamed fat around diverticula may be seen. US may detect abscess formation, although this may not be visible if the abscess contains a lot of gas, or is deep in the pelvis.

### MRI

Use is limited due to bowel movement and poor spatial resolution.

*Protocol*
T2 FS axial or coronal. T1 images post contrast enhancement will help identify abscesses.

*Findings*
- High signal on T2 around the inflamed diverticula
- Abscess formation will show an enhancing wall around a fluid-filled cavity (high signal on T2, low signal on T1)

## Differential diagnosis

- Colonic tumour: sigmoid diverticulitis can be difficult to distinguish from a colonic tumour. Factors in favour of tumour include lymph nodes in mesentery, a short segment, and intraluminal nodularity. Fluid in the mesentery and a long segment of involvement favour benign diverticulitis.
- Epiploic appendagitis: an epiploic appendage is a grape-like protusion of pericolic fat. Torsion of this can lead to infarction and inflammation, with a benign prognosis. On CT, inflammation is limited to a single fat-containing pericolic lesion, Fig 7.2a.

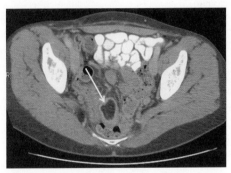

**Fig. 7.2a** Epiploic appendagitis. The epiploic appendage is seen as a fat attenuation lesion adjacent to the colon with higher attenuation surrounding inflammation.

## Management

- Conservative; fluid resuscitation and intravenous antibiotics
- Associated abscesses can usually be drained percutaneously using radiological guidance (📖 see p. 378).
- Surgery is indicated for perforated disease or failure of conservative/percutaneous management

## Complications

### To demonstrate a suspected colovesical fistula

Although CT with rectal contrast is probably the most useful investigation, either a water-soluble contrast enema or a cystogram may also be performed. On CT, look for an intimate association between the colon involved with diverticular disease and the bladder; gas in a bladder that has not been recently catheterized; and passage of rectal contrast into the bladder. CT is the most useful investigation as if there is a clear layer of normal fat between bowel and bladder, then a fistula may be excluded.

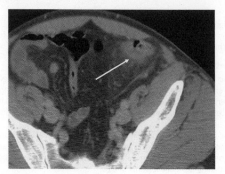

**Fig. 7.2b** Acute diverticulitis on CT. There are inflammatory changes in the surrounding fat (arrow).

**Further reading**
1. Thoeni RF and Cello JP (2006) CT imaging of colitis. *Radiology* **240**; 623–38.

# ! ? Small bowel obstruction

## Definition
Obstruction of the lumen of the small bowel.

## Aetiology and epidemiology
Small bowel obstruction (SBO) is most commonly due to hernia or adhesional disease. Other causes include Crohn's disease, gallstone ileus, volvulus from malrotation, inflamed Meckel's diverticulum, appendicitis, tumour (primary small bowel tumours are rare, metastases especially melanoma or peritoneal deposits are more common), intussusception.

## Clinical features
Vomiting, colicky abdominal pain, abdominal distension.

## Imaging
### Radiographs
Dilated, gas-filled loops of small bowel greater than 3.5cm for proximal small bowel and 2.5cm for ileum. The small bowel has folds that extend across the whole bowel wall (valvulae conniventes), in contrast to the large bowel. If the bowel loops are predominantly fluid-filled then they may not be visible. The small and large bowel will be collapsed below the level of high grade obstruction. Examine hernial orifices. Look for free gas indicating perforation, and calcified gallstones.

### Ultrasound
If history and plain film suggest SBO, then generally a CT is indicated. US may reveal an unsuspected diagnosis of SBO, or may be of use in making this diagnosis in children/young adults, especially if intussusception is the cause.

#### Protocol
General abdominal and pelvic examination using 4–6MHz curvilinear probe. Run the probe over the whole abdomen and pelvis in vertical lines starting at one side and working to the other.

#### Findings
Dilated, fluid-filled bowel loops with vigorous but non-effective peristalsis ('to-and-fro' motion of contents). If obstruction is established, however, then the bowel may become atonic. Examine hernial orifices.

### CT
#### Protocol
• Coverage from diaphragm to pubic symphysis
• No oral contrast (this would not be tolerated by these patients)
• 2.5mm reconstructions or thinner
• 100–150ml IV contrast injected at 3–4ml/s, with image acquisition at 40–60s

#### Findings
Dilated loops of small bowel greater than 3.5cm for proximal small bowel, and 2.5cm for ileum. The loops may be filled with gas, fluid or both. *The small bowel faeces sign* (Fig 7.3) indicates luminal contents that have a

speckled appearance like large bowel contents. This is associated with SBO, but is not specific.[1] Look for a 'transition point' between dilated and collapsed bowel. If there is no apparent abnormality at this point, then the cause is assumed to be adhesions. A small volume of ascites is commonly associated. Look for signs of bowel ischaemia (📖 p. 160) or perforation.

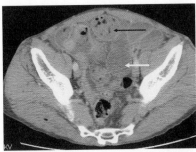

**Fig. 7.3** CT image of adhesional small bowel obstruction. Small bowel contents usually contain fluid that does not have gas bubbles within it (white arrow), but obstructed small bowel may show contents that have gas bubbles mixed within the fluid, similar to colonic contents (black arrow).

### *Barium follow-through or small bowel enema*

This should generally be avoided in the emergency setting, because barium may take a very long time to reach the level of obstruction, the patient is likely to vomit a significant amount of it, and dilution by fluid within the lumen will limit interpretation. In cases where the diagnosis of SBO is strongly suspected from plain films/CT but it is unclear whether conservative management will be successful, a modified technique is described below.

#### *Protocol*

The patient drinks 100ml Gastrografin® (diatrizoate meglumine, Schering) and plain abdominal films are taken at 1h and 4h. If contrast has not reached the colon at four hours then this suggests high grade SBO requiring surgical management.[2] Gastrografin® has a very high osmolarity and will draw fluid into the bowel which may have a therapeutic effect for low grade adhesions.

### Differential diagnosis

- Ileus: this is the most important differential, and can be difficult to distinguish from true obstruction.
- In a patient with pancreatitis, localised ileus of the small bowel can occur in the central upper abdomen, causing a 'sentinel loop' on a plain abdominal film.
- Gastric perforation.
- Gastritis.
- Cholecystitis.

**Management**

'Drip and suck': intravenous fluids and decompression of bowel via nasogastric tube.

High grade obstruction will usually require surgery but low grade can be managed conservatively (at least acutely).

# Gallstone ileus

Chronic cholecystitis causes a loop of small bowel to become adherent to the gallbladder, and a fistula forms allowing passage of a calculus. This may pass out of the bowel, or become stuck in the distal ileum (the narrowest part) causing obstruction. The calculus may be visible on plain film, as may gas in the gallbladder or biliary tree.

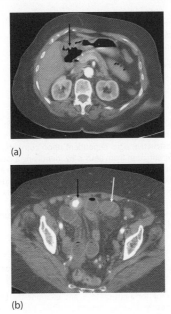

(a)

(b)

**Fig. 7.4** Gallstone ileus. (a) Abdominal CT demonstrating a gas-filled fistula between duodenum and gallbladder (arrow). (b) Calcified gallstone impacted in distal small bowel (black arrow) with dilated proximal bowel (white arrow).

**Further reading**
**1.** Mayo-Smith WW, Wittenberg J, Bennett GL *et al.* (1995) The CT small bowel faeces sign: description and clinical significance. *Clinical Radiology* **50**; 765–67.

**2.** Joyce WP, Delaney PV, Gorey TF *et al.* (1992) The value of water-soluble contrast radiology in the management of acute small bowel obstruction. *Ann R Coll Surg Engl* **74**; 422–5.

# ① ⑦ **Large bowel obstruction**

## Definition
Luminal obstruction of the large bowel.

## Aetiology and epidemiology
- Hernias
- Tumour
- Volvulus (📖 p. 164)
- Diverticular stricture
- Crohn's disease
- Intussusception

## Clinical features and differential diagnosis
As for SBO.

## Imaging
### Radiographs
The key sign is dilatation of large bowel with gas and/or fluid down to the level of obstruction. Small bowel may be normal initially, but will eventually also show obstructive signs dependent upon competence of the ileo-caecal valve. Differentiation from ileus is by identifying a clear cut-off level. If there is no such cut-off then ileus is most likely, although a very low level of obstruction (i.e. low rectum or anus) should be considered. Ileus and bowel obstruction can be difficult to differentiate and early repeat imaging is often indicated.

A colonic diameter of 6cm or greater (10cm for caecum) is abnormal and is considered a risk for perforation.

### CT
*Protocol*
No oral contrast 2.5–5mm reconstructions, post IV contrast 60s.

*Findings*
As on plain film, look for a cut-off level and examine the bowel closely at that point. A smoothly tapering pseudotransition point (Fig. 7.5) is often seen with ileus, and should not be mistaken for adhesions. Look for evidence of bowel infarction (📖 p. 160) or perforation.

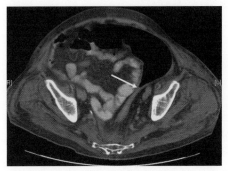

**Fig. 7.5** A smooth, tapering appearance of dependant colon (arrow) is seen in ileus, and does not represent a transition point of obstructed bowel.

### Contrast enema

This is usually reserved for clarifying the CT result in borderline cases. Most practitioners of colonic stenting appreciate a pre-procedure contrast enema to aid in clarifying the position, length and degree of tightness of a stricture.

The aim of the examination is to get contrast into a distended segment of colon, i.e. one that is above the potential level of obstruction.

#### Protocol

Since the bowel distal to the obstruction is usually empty, no bowel preparation is required. 100–500ml water soluble contrast (e.g. diatrizoate meglumine, Gastrografin®, Schering, UK; diluted 50% with water) and introduced into the rectum via a 12 Fr foley catheter and bladder syringe while the patient is in the left lateral position. Air may also be introduced to aid retrograde passage of contrast. If the level of the obstruction is above the rectosigmoid, the patient should be rolled prone to encourage contrast to pass proximally. It can be difficult to get contrast into the right colon.

#### Findings

If contrast passes freely into gas/fluid distended colon without a demonstrable stricture, then the diagnosis is pseudo-obstruction/ileus. A tapering appearance is seen with volvulus (Fig 7.6) (□ p. 164), and there is generally a delay in passage through a tumour with associated luminal narrowing and mucosal irregularity.

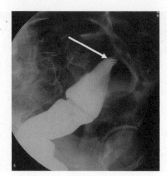

**Fig. 7.6** Beaked appearance of sigmoid volvulus at contrast enema (arrow).

*Ultrasound*
The large amount of gas present in the large bowel limits the utility of ultrasound. Occasionally when the colon is predominantly fluid-filled, and there is a clear transition point, it may be possible to make the diagnosis. However, CT is still indicated.

*MRI*
Poor spatial resolution and movement artefact limits the usefulness of MRI for investigation of the large bowel.

**Management**
Depends on cause.
- Generally, fluid resuscitation and proceed to surgery.
- A radiologically placed colonic stent can be used as the definitive management for metastatic tumour or as a bridge to surgery for a potentially curable tumour or a benign stricture. Perforation or right-sided lesions are a contraindication.

**Further reading**
**1.** Moore CJ, Corl FM, Fishman EK (2001) CT of cecal volvulus: unravelling the image. *AJR* **177**; 95–8.

**2.** Sinha R and Verma R (2005) Multidetector row computed tomography in bowel obstruction. *Clinical Radiology* **60**; 1068–75.

# ! Ischaemic bowel

### Definition
Ischaemia/hypoxia of the bowel. Mild ischaemia can be reversible, severe ischaemia results in necrosis and perforation of the bowel with a high mortality.

### Aetiology and epidemiology
The causes are many, but all causes are more common in the elderly and are less well-tolerated:
- *Luminal*: bowel obstruction causes increased intraluminal pressure which impedes blood flow.
- *Small and medium arteries*: vasculitis.
- *Large arteries*:
  - Atherosclerosis.
  - Thromboembolic disease.
  - Traumatic avulsion of vascular pedicle.
  - Iatrogenic: deliberate embolization to treat haemorrhage.
  - Aortic dissection or aneurysm repair.
- *Venous*:
  - Portal hypertension or portal venous/SMV thrombosis.
  - Volvulus or strangulated hernia: both arteries and veins are compressed, but venous system is lower pressure and is compromised first.
- *Systemic*: systemic hypotension or hypoxia. This tends to affect the watershed areas, most notably the 'Griffith point' near the splenic flexure, and the 'point of Sudek' at the rectosigmoid junction.

### Clinical features
Exact presentation depends upon the cause, but the clinical features are usually vague and non-specific. Central abdominal pain is usual, but is not severe. Inflammatory markers are raised but not dramatically so.

### Imaging
#### CT
CECT is the best modality for evaluating ischemia

##### Protocol
A standard abdomino-pelvic study will usually be performed as the diagnosis may not specifically be suspected. However, if ischaemia is specifically being investigated the optimal technique is:
- No oral contrast or oral water if tolerated
- Consider NECT at 5mm resolution look for intramural haemorrhage.
- Late arterial phase at high resolution: 40s; 2.5mm or thinner.
- Consider portal venous phase to reliably assess the liver.

##### Findings
- Ischaemia most commonly affects left colon.
- The most important sign is segmental failure of bowel wall enhancement.
- High attenuation material in the bowel wall on an unenhanced scan indicates intramural haemorrhage.

- The bowel wall may be thickened or thinned, may be hyper- or hypoattenuating, and may be non-enhancing or hyperenhancing (the latter is difficult to distinguish from haemorrhage if a NECT was not performed).
- Normal bowel wall is 3–6mm thick, but this must be interpreted in the light of the amount of luminal distension. In a well distended segment of large or small bowel the wall is almost imperceptibly thin.
- Examine coeliac, superior and inferior mesenteric arteries and corresponding veins for thrombus or luminal narrowing or, if there is a traumatic aetiology, complete disruption. Appreciation of the latter may be aided by sagittal reformats.
- Venous infarction causes gross oedema due to congestion.
- Mild reversible ischaemia causes a hyperenhancing thickened bowel wall, whereas arterio-occlusive infarction causes a non-enhancing, paper-thin bowel wall, in a dilated segment of bowel.
- Other than direct visualization of arterial thrombus, all other signs such as mesenteric fat stranding, ascites and the 'target sign', Fig. 7.7a (enhancement of muscularis and mucosa, with oedema of submucosa) are non-specific.
- Gas in the mesenteric veins or portal vein usually indicates severe ischaemia of the bowel wall. However, portomesenteric gas may be seen from other, benign causes (see differential below).[1] Within the liver portal venous gas is distinguished from biliary gas in that it reaches the periphery of the liver.
- Gas in the bowel wall may be confused with intraluminal gas bubbles seen in ileus.
- Free gas indicates bowel perforation.
- Associated infarcts in other organs (e.g. kidneys, spleen) may be seen.

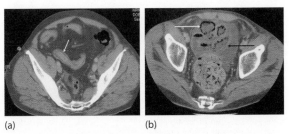

(a)  (b)

**Fig. 7.7** (a) 'Target sign'—enhancement of muscularis and mucosa, with oedema of submucosa. (b) Necrotic small bowel shows intramural gas, and non-enhancement of the bowel wall (white arrow). Other pelvic small bowel loops show enhancement and wall thickening (black arrow).

### Differential diagnosis

For ischaemic colitis, the differential includes most other causes of colitis. The gross wall thickening seen in venous infarction is also seen in pseudomembranous colitis.

Portomesenteric venous gas is also seen in gastric ulceration, inflammatory bowel disease, after procedures which distend the bowel (e.g. CT colonography) and occasionally with diverticulitis and ileus.[1]

## Management

Many cases of bowel ischaemia are reversible, and conservative management is appropriate. For cases of bowel infarction assessment at laparotomy and resection of infarcted bowel is required.

**Further reading**
**1.** Sebastià C, Quiroga S, Espin E et al. (2000) Portomesenteric vein gas: pathologic mechanisms, CT findings, and prognosis. *Radiographics* **20**; 1213–24, discussion 1224–6.

# ⚠ Volvulus

## Definition

A volvulus is twisting of a loop of bowel on its mesentery, causing luminal obstruction and vascular compromise. Since the bowel lumen is obstructed at two points, it is termed a 'closed loop obstruction'. Any form of obstruction will progress to necrosis and perforation of the affected bowel eventually.

## Clinical features

Sudden onset pain and bowel obstruction. May be recurrent, with spontaneous resolution

## Imaging

### Radiographs

A plain film may be diagnostic for sigmoid volvulus, but for all other volvuli, a CT is required for diagnosis.

### Contrast enema

*Protocol*
📖 p. 157 for details (LBO).

### CT

*Protocol*
📖 p. 152.

*Findings*

The two limbs of the volvulus gradually taper and converge at the site of the torsion. The mesenteric vessels should show a marked twisting or 'whorl'. In all voluli, look for signs of bowel ischaemia or perforation (see 📖 p. 160 and p. 168).

## Classification

### Gastric volvulus

This is rare and usually associated with a hiatus hernia. If the stomach is twisted along its long axis (organoaxial) this is associated with more complications (obstruction and ischaemia) than if it rotates along its short axis (mesenteroaxial).

### Small bowel volvulus (SMV)

This occurs mainly in association with malrotation. The root of the small bowel mesentery is narrower than normal, allowing the small bowel to rotate. AXR may show dilated loops of small bowel, possibly with gastric dilatation. CT will show central dilated small bowel loops. The small bowel vessels show a whorled appearance. Signs of malrotation are an abnormal relationship between the superior mesenteric arteries and veins (vein normally lies to the right of the artery) and an abnormal position of the duodenojejunal flexure (should be at the level of L1, to the left of the spine).

### Caecal volvulus

The caecal pole either spins on its axis, remaining in the right iliac fossa, or flips upward to lie centrally. AXR will show a large gas-filled viscus representing the caecum either centrally or in the right iliac fossa. Small bowel obstruction will develop proximally. The diagnosis is confirmed by CT. Visualization of the appendix is useful to locate the caecal pole. A third variant a 'caecal bascule' occurs when the caecum folds anteriorly without torsion.[1]

### Sigmoid volvulus

The sigmoid colon rotates on its mesenteric axis. This is associated with a large, tortuous colon.

AXR can be diagnostic:

- *Coffee bean sign*: the huge gas-distended loop of sigmoid colon is oval in shape and generally ahaustral but with a prominent fold at the left lower edge which resembles a coffee bean, Fig 7.8.
- *Left iliac fossa convergence* of the distended bowel loop.
- *Left flank overlap sign*: the left margin of the bowel loop overlaps the descending colon.
- Apex of loop above level of T10.
- Gas: fluid ratio of >2:1; i.e. the volved segment contains mostly gas.
- Large bowel obstruction above the level of the volvulus.

CT will show the typical features of a volvulus centred upon the sigmoid mesocolon, with large bowel obstruction proximally.

Contrast enema shows a classic tapering beaked appearance which is seen at the lower level of obstruction (Fig 7.6).

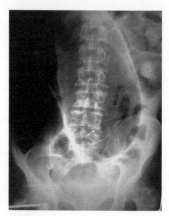

**Fig. 7.8** Plain abdominal film showing 'coffee bean' sign of sigimoid volvulus.

**Differential diagnosis**
Other causes of bowel obstruction.

**Further reading**

**1.** Moore CJ, Corl FM and Fishman EK (2001) CT of cecal volvulus: unraveling the image. *AJR* **177**; 95–8.

# ⓘ **Bowel perforation**

## Definition

Bowel perforation indicates a hole somewhere in the GI tract allowing bowel contents (gas, liquid or solid) to pass in to the mediastinum, peritoneum or retroperitoneum. This is usually an emergency requiring surgical intervention.

The hallmark of perforation is therefore gas outside the bowel lumen. In the case of an oesophageal perforation this will be within the mediastinum. Perforation of stomach and small bowel usually results in peritoneal free gas. Perforation of the third part of the duodenum or rectum usually results in retroperitoneal free gas. Perforation of other structures may result in peritoneal or retroperitoneal free gas. Remember that free gas is to be expected after a laparotomy, and may persist for up to 2 weeks.

## Aetiology

- Gastric or duodenal perforation secondary to ulceration.
- Sigmoid diverticulitis.
- Iatrogenic: usually endoscopic procedures.
- Traumatic.
- Secondary to obstructed or ischaemic bowel.
- Perforated tumour, especially colonic.
- Appendicitis.

The most common causes of bowel perforation are duodenal or gastric ulceration and sigmoid diverticular disease. It is not uncommon for large amounts of gas but very little faeces to be released from a sigmoid colon perforation and this has a good prognosis with conservative management.

## Imaging

### Radiographs

*Protocol*

The erect CXR is the best initial test, and gas is identified under the diaphragm. The patient must sit up for at least 10min to allow gas to percolate through the abdomen.

Patients who cannot tolerate erect CXR examinations could have standard abdominal films. A better alternative is either a left lateral decubitus or a lateral shoot-through (the patient is supine and the X-ray beam is directed laterally through the abdomen).

*Findings*

Tiny amounts of gas can be detected using an erect CXR[1], but only 70% of perforations will show free gas with this technique. Care must be taken to distinguish luminal gas in stomach or colon from free gas:

- Look carefully for haustral or rugal markings in the candidate gas pocket.
- If a gastric gas bubble is not seen separate to the candidate gas pocket under the left hemidiaphragm, then it probably is the stomach.
- Look for gas outlining the falciform ligament.
- Sometimes basal linear atelectasis or basal bullae may mimic free gas.
- Free gas pockets are often triangular, whereas intraluminal gas has curvilinear margins.

- *Rigler's sign*: gas on either side of the bowel wall. The gas must be as 'black' outside the wall as it is inside—do not mistake the relative lucency of mesenteric fat for free gas.

Bear in mind that it is not always possible to make the diagnosis with plain films and in sick patients, CT should be performed without delay.

## CT

*Protocol*

- Coverage from diaphragm to pubic symphysis.
- Oral contrast medium 20min prior to study.
- 2.5 or 5mm reconstructions.
- IV contrast medium at 60s.

The technique could be modified according to the most likely suspected underlying diagnosis.

*Findings*

Examine the entire data set slowly on lung windows looking for triangular gas shadows outside the bowel wall. Remember to examine the retroperitoneum, where gas pockets tend to be irregular rather than triangular. If there is free gas, there will usually be free fluid as well. The site with the largest collection of free gas usually indicates the point of underlying pathology, although gas can move anteriorly and superiorly. Look for an obvious defect in the bowel wall.

## Management

This depends upon the underlying diagnosis, but will usually be surgical.

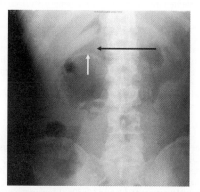

**Fig. 7.9** AXR showing a large triangular collection of free gas (black arrow) and gas on either side of the bowel wall (Rigler's sign, white arrow).

## Further reading

**1.** Miller RE and Nelson SW (1971) The roentgenologic demonstration of tiny amounts of free intraperitoneal gas: experimental and clinical studies. *Am J Roentgenol Radium Ther Nucl Med* **112**(3); 574–85.

# ⚠ ⚕ Cholecystitis and cholangitis

## Definition and aetiology

Cholecystitis is inflammation of the gallbladder and in the majority of cases is associated with calculi.

Cholangitis is infection of the bile ducts and is usually associated with blockage of the ducts secondary to calculi (rarely with malignant obstruction) or with reflux of bile contents into the ducts from previous surgery or sphincterotomy. Cholangitis is also associated with diabetes. Liver abscesses may develop.

## Clinical features

Right upper quadrant pain, signs of sepsis, abnormal liver function tests.

## Imaging

### Ultrasound

Ultrasound is the definitive examination.

*Protocol*

General abdominal examination using 3–6MHz curvilinear probe. Patients should be fasted for 4hrs.

*Findings*

Look for thickening of the gallbladder wall (>3mm), calculi, pericholecystic fluid, tenderness over the gallbladder or an enlarged gallbladder.

Gas in the gallbladder may be due to reflux of gas from the duodenum, or may be generated from bacterial growth (emphysematous cholecystitis). This is commoner in people with diabetes and has a worse prognosis.

There is no universal agreement for the upper limit of normal of the common bile duct or whether it may be dilated after cholecystectomy, but most authors use 6mm. The intrahepatic bile ducts should not be more than a third of the diameter of the accompanying portal vein branch. Air in the biliary tree (pneumobilia) is seen as brightly echogenic lines replacing the intrahepatic bile ducts, with dense posterior shadowing.

The main limitation of ultrasound is that the distal CBD is often not seen. MRCP is the best test to examine this region.

### CT

*Protocol*

- Oral water (not oral contrast as this may obscure a calculus in the distal CBD).
- A NECT examination with 5mm or thinner slice thickness is essential for maximal sensitivity in detecting a subtle ductal calculus.
- Images post IV contrast at 40s and 60–70s, slice thickness: 2.5mm or less.

*Findings*

As for ultrasound (see above). Biliary calculi may have a range of densities on CT ranging from less than water (some calculi have gas within them) to the very high density of calcified calculi. 80% are cholesterol or of mixed composition and 20% are pigment stones (primarily calcium bilirubinate). A significant minority are of such similar density to water (bile) that they are essentially invisible.

Hepatic abscesses will be low attenuation with avidly enhancing walls.

## MRCP

*Protocol*

The cornerstone of magnetic resonance cholangiopancreatography (MRCP) is heavily T2-weighted fat suppressed images. Signal is only retained from stationary fluid, i.e. bile. Thick (usually 10–20mm) MIP images are recon-structed at varying angles centred around the CBD and thin slices (1–2mm) should also be available for comparison. Coronal and axial T1 and T2 images should also be performed. Contrast is generally not necessary (Fig 7.10).

*Findings*

As for ultrasound (see above). Biliary calculi have no signal on MRI. It is normal to sometimes see a low signal line running down the centre of the duct. This is a flow artefact and should not be mistaken for calculi.
Hepatic abscesses will be high signal on T2 and low signal on T1, and are difficult to distinguish from metastases or haemangiomas without admin-istering IV contrast.

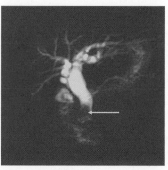

**Fig.7.10** MIP image from an MRCP showing a grossly dilated biliary tree with a large obstructing calculus in the distal CBD (arrow).

**Is a biliary stent patent?**

Even after relief of biliary obstruction, the biliary tree may remain dilated. If the patient has a biliary stent *in situ*, gas in the bile ducts indicates patency of the stent. However, absence of gas does not necessarily mean blockage. Pneumobilia can be seen easily on CT or US, but is harder to perceive on MRI.

**Management**

Cholecystitis is traditionally managed by antibiotic therapy and analgesia followed by cholecystectomy in the convalescent period, although surgical trends are now toward early surgery. Failure to respond to conservative management may necessitate an early cholecystostomy or placement of a percutaneous catheter in the gallbladder under image guidance.

Sepsis associated with a bile duct calculus should be treated by removal of the calculus at ERCP. If the calculus cannot be removed, it can be bypassed by a stent deployed either at ERCP or percutaneously.

# ! ? **Pancreatitis**

Inflammation of the pancreas.

## Aetiology

- Obstruction of pancreatic duct by biliary calculi.
- Alcohol.
- Iatrogenic, especially after ERCP procedures.
- Drugs.
- Tumours.

## Clinical features

Pain, vomiting, sepsis. The diagnosis is usually based upon a history and a raised serum amylase, but CT imaging is increasingly used in uncertain cases.

## Imaging

All patients with pancreatitis should have imaging of the biliary tree with US, although this does not need to be done as an emergency unless the liver function tests are abnormal. CT examination is not routinely indicated, although is increasingly being used.[1]

### *Ultrasound*

*Protocol*

General abdominal examination using 3–6MHz curvilinear probe.

*Findings*

The pancreas may be diffusely hypoechoic indicating inflammation, or may appear normal. It is common not to be able to see the pancreas due to overlying bowel gas. Look for fluid collections anywhere within the abdomen or pelvis. Pleural effusions are commonly associated. Examination of the biliary tree is critical. Look for dilated bile ducts (CBD >6mm). Look for calculi both within the gallbladder and within the ducts. It is common for the distal CBD not to be visualized, indicating the need for an MRCP or ERCP.

### *CT*

*Protocol*

- Oral water (not oral contrast as this may obscure a calculus in the distal CBD).
- A NECT examination with 5mm or thinner slice thickness is essential for maximal sensitivity in detecting a subtle ductal calculus.
- Images post IV contrast at:
  - 40s; 2.5mm or thinner through pancreas; small field of view
  - 60–70s; 5mm or thinner; whole abdomen and pelvis.

*Findings*

The hallmark of pancreatitis is high attenuation stranding in the peripancreatic fat. This may be associated with increased size and reduced attenuation of the gland and peripancreatic fluid. The upper limit of normal for the pancreatic duct is 3mm within the pancreatic head; it should taper towards the tail.

The pre-contrast examination is to detect calculi in the biliary tree, although a significant minority will be invisible on CT. It will also demonstrate haemorrhage within the pancreas or within peripancreatic fluid collections. The presence of pancreatic calcification indicates chronic pancreatitis.

The pancreatic phase (40s) is to assess the pancreas for viability (dead pancreas does not enhance) and also to detect tumours that may have precipitated the inflammation.

The portal venous phase is to assess complications such as portal vein or splenic vein thrombosis, peripancreatic fluid collections (those still present 1 month after the onset of symptoms are termed pseudocysts) and local or distant abscesses.

### MRCP

Used to assess the biliary tree for intraductal calculi not seen on other imaging modalities.

#### Protocol

As for cholecystitis/cholangitis ( p. 170). Axial T1 fat suppressed (FS) images are useful for assessing chronic pancreatitis: a normal pancreas is very high signal on this sequence, but this signal is reduced in chronic pancreatitis.

#### Findings

Calculi have no signal, and careful examination of the thin T2 FS images is required. It is normal to sometimes see a low signal line running down the centre of the duct. This is a flow artefact and should not be mistaken for calculi.

Also assess the pancreatic duct for obstruction by tumour, calculi, and for signs of chronic pancreatitis (dilatation of the main duct—which is normally up to 3mm in the head—and side branches; irregularity of the main duct.)

### Differential diagnosis

- Biliary colic
- Cholecystitis
- Gastritis
- Gastric perforation
- Small bowel obstruction

### Management

Obstructing biliary calculi should be sought and removed. Management is otherwise supportive with drainage of infected fluid collections using percutaneous drains placed under image guidance.[1]

### Further reading

1. UK Working Party on Acute Pancreatitis (2005) UK guidelines for the management of acute pancreatitis. *Gut* 54(Suppl III); iii1–iii9. Available at http://www.gut.bmj.com/cgi/content/extract/54/suppl_3/iii1.

# ① ⑦ Colitis

### Definition
Inflammation of the colon.

### Aetiology
- Ulcerative colitis and Crohn's disease
- Infective:
  - Pseudomembranous colitis; infection with *Clostridium difficile* is endemic in UK hospitals
  - CMV (associated with immunosuppression)
  - Amoebic (associated with foreign travel)
  - Tuberculous
- Ischaemic, especially secondary to tumour
- Idiopathic

### Clinical features
Diarrhoea, abdominal pain, fever, tenesmus, blood per rectum (PR).

### Imaging
CT, plain films and sometimes US can be used to determine the extent of colitis in patients in whom full endoscopy is considered too risky. CT colonography (pneumocolon) or barium enema should not be performed in patients with acute colitis because of the risk of bowel perforation.

#### Radiographs: AXR
In an ill patient with suspected acute colitis, a plain film is mandatory to exclude toxic megacolon. In hospitalized patients, serial imaging is often required.

*Findings*
- Toxic megacolon:
  - dilatation of colon greater than 6cm, except the caecum which can be up to 10cm
- Perforation (on erect CXR if possible)

#### CT
CT imaging is not generally necessary for the diagnosis or management of colitis. It may be used in cases of undiagnosed abdominal pain and diarrhoea.

In patients with known colitis who have deteriorated, CT can be used to diagnose complications such as perforation or abscess formation.

*Protocol*
- Coverage from diaphragm to pubic symphysis
- Oral contrast medium 20min prior to study
- 5mm reconstructions or thinner
- 100–150ml IV contrast at 3–4ml/s, with image acquisition at 60s

*Findings*
*Target sign:* a thickened bowel wall with avid enhancement of the mucosa and muscularis, contrasting with oedema and reduced enhancement of the sub-mucosa. This is a useful sign as it rarely occurs with malignancy. It should be distinguished from the *fat halo sign* where fat is deposited in the submucosa in chronic inflammatory bowel disease, and occasionally in normal patients.[1]

The *comb sign* describes engorged vascular mesentery, and although usually attributed to Crohn's disease, is non-specific.

**Features suggesting the cause of colitis**

1. Concurrent small bowel disease is seen in backwash ileitis (inflammation of the last few centimetres of the terminal ileum) of *ulcerative colitis*, terminal ileal stricturing in *tuberculosis*, and more diffuse disease in *Crohn's disease*.

2. *Crohn's disease:* skip lesions, small bowel disease, fistula formation including perianal region.

3. *Ulcerative colitis:* continuous disease spreading retrogradely from the anus, although a caecal patch can also occur. Backwash ileitis. Rectal sparing can occur.

4. *Tuberculosis:* conical narrowing of the caecum associated with terminal ileal strictures and caseating lymph nodes.

5. *CMV* tends to be right-sided in immunocompromised patients, although can complicate ulcerative colitis in which case it will be left-sided.

6. Massive colonic wall thickening (more than 1cm, sometimes over 2cm) with lack of a 'halo' sign is most suggestive of *pseudomembranous colitis* (infection by *Clostridium difficile*). The grossly thickened haustra pressed together produce the *accordion sign*, Fig 7.11. This is a common cause of colitis in hospitalized patients[2] and is usually a pancolitis, although rectal and sigmoid sparing can occur.

7. *Ischaemic colitis:* distribution may be segmental, often sparing the rectum or may be limited to the watershed areas. There may be associated vascular disease (see 📖 p. 160).

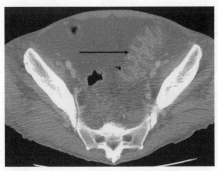

**Fig. 7.11** *Accordion sign* (arrow) in *Clostridium difficile* colitis. There is also a large amount of ascites.

## Further reading

**1.** Amitai MM, Arazi-Kleinman T, Avidan B *et al.* (2007) Fat halo sign in the bowel wall of patients with Crohn's disease. *Clin Radiol* **62**; 994–7.

**2.** Fishman EK, Kavuru M, Jones B *et al.* (1991) Pseudomembranous colitis: CT evaluation of 26 cases. *Radiology* **180**; 57–60.

# ① ⑦ **Abdominal collection**

### Definition
A collection of pus within the abdomen or pelvis.

### Aetiology
Many causes including: appendicitis, diverticular disease, Crohn's disease and post-operative.

### Clinical features
Abdominal pain, fever, sepsis, localized tenderness, diarrhoea.

### Imaging
US should be the first-line investigation in young people. However, retroperitoneal or deep pelvic abscesses may not be visible. US is especially limited in post-operative patients who have wounds, stomas, drains and dressings limiting the sonographic windows. Early transfer to CT is advised. MRI is generally useful, but is often not possible in the post-operative period due to use of surgical clips.

#### *Ultrasound*
*Protocol*
General abdominal and pelvic examination using 4–6MHz curvilinear probe. Run the probe over the whole abdomen and pelvis in vertical lines starting at one side and working to the other.

*Findings*
An abscess will generally be hypoechoic with thick walls. It is often tender. Abscesses may be echogenic or have prominent septa within them.

#### *CT*
*Protocol*
- Coverage from diaphragm to pubic symphysis
- Oral contrast medium at least 20min prior to study
- 5mm reconstructions or thinner
- 100–150ml IV contrast at 3–4 ml/s, with image acquisition at 60s

*Findings*
An abscess will usually be of fluid attenuation with thick, usually enhancing walls.

#### *MRI*
*Protocol*
Axial and coronal T1 and T2, fat-suppressed T1 images pre and post IV contrast for abdomen and pelvis. Sagittal T2 sequences for pelvis.

*Findings*
An abscess will be high signal on T2, and usually low signal on T1. There is usually no enhancement of the central contents and a thick, enhancing wall.

### General considerations

Care should always be taken to differentiate an abscess from abnormal bowel. Dilated, aperistaltic bowel can easily be mistaken for an abscess. CT, with its higher spatial resolution and with use of oral contrast, is the most reliable test to differentiate the two.

When reporting abscesses, comment should be made as to the possibility and ease of percutaneous drainage.

### Management

Image guided aspiration and drainage is covered in the interventional section (📖 p. 378).

### Further reading

1. Maher MM, Gervais DA, Kalra MK et al. (2004) The inaccessible or undrainable abscess: how to drain it. Radiographics 24(3); 717–35.

# ! Oesophageal rupture

## Aetiology
- Iatrogenic from diagnostic endoscopy or from dilatation of a tumour or of achalasia.
- Spontaneous from vomiting (Boerhaave syndrome).
- Perforation of a tumour.

## Clinical features
Acute chest pain, haematemesis, fever.

## Imaging

### Radiographs
This diagnosis should be considered in the presence of any mediastinal gas. Pleural effusions and pneumothoraces are common, but non-specific.

### Contrast swallow

*Protocol*
Water-soluble contrast media (WSCM) should be used. Any agent with an iodine concentration of 300mg/l is acceptable apart from diatrizoate meglumine (Gastrografin®) which has a high osmolarity. If this is accidentally aspirated, it can draw water into the lungs, causing pulmonary oedema. In general, barium should not be used although some practitioners may give barium after a normal examination with WSCM, arguing that barium is denser and therefore more sensitive for small perforations. Although a large amount of barium in the mediastinum is undesirable, small amounts appear to be safe.[1]

The patient should be examined semi-supine (20°) on the fluoroscopy table and water-soluble contrast should be given in the cup with a straw. Boluses of contrast are followed down the oesophagus into the stomach, and then this is repeated in the left and right lateral positions.

*Findings*
A perforation is diagnosed when an irregular pool of contrast is seen outside of the lumen. Look for irregular mucosal strictures indicating a tumour.

### CT

*Protocol*
- Coverage to include chest and upper abdomen.
- Oral contrast medium 20min prior to the study.
- 5 mm reconstructions or thinner.
- 100–150ml IV contrast at 3–4ml/s, with image acquisition at 25–60s.

*Findings*
Although CT is not the best test for diagnosing a perforation, it may be used in patients with chest pain and plain film signs suggestive of the diagnosis where there is a wide differential diagnosis.

Occasionally the oesophageal perforation will be directly visualised, but more often it is suggested by gas and fluid collections in the mediastinum. Pleural effusions and pneumothoraces are associated.

## Differential diagnosis
- Oesophageal apoplexy
- Myocardial infarction
- Aortic dissection

## Further reading
**1.** James AE Jr, Montali RJ, Chaffee V *et al.* (1975) Barium or gastrografin: which contrast media for diagnosis of esophageal tears? *Gastroenterology* **68**; 1103–13.

# ① ⑦ Acute liver failure

## Imaging

Imaging has a limited role in acute liver failure and is used mainly in aiding prognosis.

### Ultrasound

*Protocol*

General abdominal examination using 3–6MHz curvilinear probe. Colour Doppler should be used to assess the hepatic artery and veins and the portal vein. Normal flow in the portal vein is toward the liver.

### CT

*Protocol*

- Oral water.
- NECT: 5mm slice thickness.
- CECT:
  - 25s; 2.5mm or thinner through whole liver.
  - 60–70s; 5mm or thinner through the whole abdomen and pelvis.

### MRI

*Protocol*

Liver imaging with MRI is outside the scope of this book, but multiphasic contrast enhancement is helpful in diagnosing hepatocellular carcinoma.

## General imaging findings

- Ascites: ultrasound may be used to guide a diagnostic ascitic tap for suspected bacterial peritonitis (see 📖 p. 378).
- Assess for patency of the portal vein and presence of portal vein/splenic vein/superior mesenteric vein thrombosis. Ultrasound is the only modality which can determine the direction of flow in the portal vein easily. Normally, blood flowing toward the probe is displayed as red, and blood flowing away as blue. If the portal vein is perpendicular to the insonating beam then Doppler signal will be poor or absent despite good flow. Absence of flow in the portal vein should be interpreted with caution as it may merely represents slow flow rather than thrombus.
- Evidence of portal hypertension: splenomegaly and collateral vessels. Look for collateral vessels in the falciform ligament, around the left kidney and at the gastro-oesophageal junction (the latter is not always visible on ultrasound).
- Hepatic vein thrombosis (Budd–Chiari syndrome) is a very rare disorder associated with hypercoaguable states. Direct visualization of thrombus is diagnostic, but this can be difficult to determine. The differential diagnosis is growth of a hepatocellular carcinoma extending along a hepatic vein, which is more common.
- Signs of cirrhosis: a small, nodular liver, with an irregular margin.
- In acute liver failure the liver will be enlarged and often show fatty infiltration.
- Enlargement of the liver is somewhat subjective, but can be diagnosed if the right lobe measures more than 15cm in the anterior axillary line, overlaps the right kidney or if the left lobe can be seen in the left flank.

- Fatty infiltration is diagnosed on ultrasound if the liver is markedly more echogenic than the right kidney when the two are on the same image. On CT, it is diagnosed when the unenhanced attenuation is 20 HU or more below that of the spleen.
- Look for focal liver lesions which may represent tumours causing acute liver failure. Acute liver failure may be caused in non-cirrhotic livers by multiple metastases.
- Hepatic artery thrombosis is a serious complication of liver transplantation, and patency of the hepatic artery should be assessed in these patients.

### Further reading

1. Baron RL and Peterson MS (2001) From the RSNA refresher courses: screening the cirrhotic liver or hepatocellular carcinoma with CT and MR imaging: opportunities and pitfalls. *RadioGraphics* 21; S117–32.

# :⚙: ① Abdominal trauma

## Overview

- Crush injuries tend to cause tears and subcapsular haematomas to solid viscera. Transient increase in the intraluminal pressure of hollow organs may cause perforation.
- Deceleration injuries cause stretching and linear shearing, damaging renal or mesenteric vessels. A hepatic tear along the ligamentum teres is also commonly seen.
- Penetrating injuries clearly may damage any organ, and usually require surgical exploration.

## Imaging

### Ultrasound

*Protocol*

Ultrasound is often used as the primary modality for assessing abdominal trauma. FAST (focused abdominal sonography in trauma) has almost replaced diagnostic peritoneal lavage as a means of rapidly assessing polytrauma patients in the emergency room.[1]

The main purpose of the examination is to look for peritoneal free fluid, which in the context of trauma is assumed to be blood. The probe is placed in four positions; both flanks, epigastrium and suprapubic region. These positions also enable detection of pericardial and pleural fluid. If the patient has a urinary catheter, this should be used to fill the bladder with 200–300ml of sterile saline. An extension of this technique involves examining the anterior superior chest wall for a pneumothorax (supine plain films are frequently obtained in such patients which are relatively insensitive for detecting pneumothoraces): lack of normal pleural sliding is strongly suggestive of this diagnosis.[2]

*Findings*

Even a tiny amount of fluid is abnormal, with the exception of pelvic fluid less than 3cm in maximum anteroposterior dimension in women of reproductive age.

Although lacerations and haematomas of the solid abdominal organs can be detected by ultrasound, this is not the purpose of the FAST scan, and ultrasound cannot exclude solid organ injury (ultrasound has a 69% sensitivity for splenic laceration[4]), bowel injury or retroperitoneal haematoma. Solid organ lacerations/haematomas can appear hypo- or hyperechoic on ultrasound, and have no flow within them.

### CT

*Protocol*

- Coverage from diaphragm to pubic symphysis.
- Either oral water or no oral contrast. (Oral contrast may obscure bowel wall haemorrhage)
- 5mm reconstructions or thinner.
- 100-150ml IV contrast at 3–4ml/s, with image acquisition at 60s.
- Non-contrast CT will show areas of haemorrhage as high attenuation areas, but this is not performed in every centre.

- Consider use of arterial phase to assess for active bleeding and arterial integrity.

## CT findings in abdominal trauma

- Look for any peritoneal fluid.
- Look for bony injuries, especially spinal. The spine should be assessed using sagittal and coronal reformatted thin section images.
- Rib fractures may indicate the site of injury and direct the radiologist towards associated visceral injuries.
- Carefully examine all solid organs for areas of decreased attenuation: either irregular lacerations or smooth, rounded subcapsular haematomas.
- Assess lung bases for pneumothorax and diaphragmatic rupture.
- Look for free gas indicating bowel injury. The third part of the duodenum is the most commonly damaged part of the intestines as blunt trauma can compress it against the spine (for the same reason the body of the pancreas is the most frequently damaged part). Examine the mesentery for damage to the vessels.
- If there is a pancreatic laceration, examine the pancreatic duct for integrity.
- High attenuation bile may indicate haemobilia, although IV contrast has delayed excretion through the biliary system.
- A collapsed gallbladder with pericholecystic fluid suggests gallbladder perforation.
- Assess IVC distension for success of intravenous fluid resuscitation.
- Liver lacerations that extend to the porta hepatis are frequently associated with bile duct injuries.
- Kidneys should be assessed for vascular avulsion.

## Management

Patients who are haemodynamically stable with a negative US scan and low clinical probability of abdominal trauma may generally be safely observed for 24hrs,[3] although the referenced study used comprehensive ultrasounds performed by sonographers rather than a FAST scan. Those with a positive FAST scan should be taken straight for exploratory laparotomy or more fully assessed with CT, depending upon the clinical condition. *Definitive management by surgery of an unstable patient should not be delayed by CT examination.* Penetrating trauma usually requires surgical exploration.

Ultrasound follow-up of splenic injuries is useful to exclude pseudoaneurysm formation.

## Further reading

**1.** Kretschmer K-H, Bohndorf K and Pohlenz O (1997) The role of sonography in abdominal trauma: the European experience. *American Society of Emergency Radiology* **2**; 62–7.

**2.** Dulchavsky SA, Schwarz KL, Kirkpatrick A *et al.* (2001) Prospective evaluation of thoracic ultrasound in the detection of pneumothorax. Journal of *Trauma–Injury Infection and Critical Care* **50**(32); 201–5.

**3.** Sirlin CB, Brown MA, Andrade-Barrato OA *et al.* (2004) Blunt abdominal truama: clinical value of negative screening US scans. *Radiology* **230**; 661–8.

**4.** Richards JR, McGahan JP, Jones CD *et al.* (2001) Ultrasound detection of blunt splenic injury. *Injury* **32**; 95–103.

# Renal

Simon Milburn

# ⓘ Bladder rupture

### Definition and aetiology

Ruptures are divided into intraperitoneal (blunt trauma to a full bladder) or more commonly, extraperitoneal (associated with pelvic fractures). Causes: blunt trauma (RTAs, falls and assaults), penetrating trauma and iatrogenic injury (pelvic surgery or intravesical instrumentation).

### Clinical features

The classic triad of haematuria, suprapubic pain/tenderness and difficulty/ inability passing urine is often not present.

### Imaging

#### Retrograde cystogram

*Protocol*

- Perform an initial retrograde urethrogram (see urethral injury).
- Control film. Slowly fill the bladder with water-soluble contrast (e.g. Urografin®) using gravity. If fluoroscopy is available screen whilst instilling, if not stop after 100ml and obtain a film to look for gross extravasation. Fill the bladder with at least 300ml. Obtain AP, oblique and post drainage films.

*Findings*

- Filling defects due to intravesical haematoma or external compression.
- Intraperitoneal tear: normally from dome; accumulates above bladder and outlines bowel.
- Extraperitoneal: irregular, streaky appearance in the perivesical fat, tracking into the abdominal wall and perineum.
- Subserosal: rare, elliptical collection adjacent to the bladder.

#### CT cystogram

*Protocol*

- Rupture may be seen on a normal CECT if delayed images are acquired but without bladder distention it has a low sensitivity.
- If suspected, the bladder can be distended as described above, the pelvis scanned and then repeated post drainage. However, this procedure should only be performed after consideration of the radiation dose to the pelvis, especially in women of child-bearing age.

*Findings*

- Extravasation of contrast and intravesical haematoma.

### Differential diagnosis

- Traumatic haematuria—urethral, ureteric or renal injury.

### Management

- Surgery for intraperitoneal tears and conservative with catheterization for extraperitoneal.

## ⚙ ⚠ **Renal trauma**

### Definition and aetiology

Most are caused by road traffic accidents.
Other causes include: falls, assaults and sports injuries.

### Epidemiology

Renal is the most common urological injury following trauma, accounting for 10% of significant abdominal injuries. 80% are due to blunt trauma and most major renal injuries are associated with other organ damage.

### Clinical features

Flank pain/bruising, haematuria, shock and lower rib fractures.

### Imaging

Deciding who needs imaging is controversial and should be agreed upon after discussion with urologists/trauma surgeons. The following indications are meant only as a guide:

- Penetrating injuries
- Frank haematuria
- Microscopic haematuria with shock
- Other signs of significant injury (rib and transverse process fractures or extensive bruising) indicate imaging.

Patients with microscopic haematuria, who are not shocked, are unlikely to have significant renal trauma and observation alone may be appropriate. Children may have microscopic haematuria associated with severe injuries in the absence of shock.

### CT

*Protocol*

There are triple (unenhanced, arterial and delayed) phase protocols specific to renal trauma but most are carried out as part of a generalized abdominal trauma scan (5mm or less slice thickness, 100ml of IV contrast at 3–4ml/s, scanned at 60s). If perinephric/ureteral fluid is seen then a delayed scan at 10–15min may demonstrate extravasation; only practical in stable patients.

*Findings*

- Following severe trauma, multiple organs may be affected and therefore all organs should be carefully assessed.
- There is a widely used classification system (AAST; see below) but the things to look for are, in approximately increasing severity:
- **Haematomas**: *Subcapsular* between parenchyma and capsule. *Small* are crescenteric in shape but *larger* bleeds can compress the parenchyma. *Perinephric* are ill-defined between Gerota's fascia and renal parenchyma. Often associated with underlying injury.
- **Lacerations**: Superficial (<1cm depth) or deep, with or without collecting system involvement (urine/contrast extravasation).
- **Segmental infarctions**: well demarcated low attenuation, wedge shaped.
- **Arterial injury**: *Division*—large haematoma. *Occlusion*—global decreased perfusion and possibly retrograde filing of the vein.

- **Venous injury**: *Division*—smaller haematoma than above.
  *Occlusion*—delayed and progressively dense nephrogram.
- **Renal pelvis**: Urinoma (density the same as urine in the bladder) with
  contrast extravasation on delayed images. If contrast is seen in the
  distal ureter it implies a partial division.
- **Shattered**: Multiple lacerations with associated haematoma and infarction.

*US*

- FAST scan may demonstrate free fluid indicating the need for
  a laparotomy. If the patient is stable, the request for a CT will
  soon follow.
- Limited use in the acute setting as it is poor at differentiating the type of
  fluid or its source, and has relatively low sensitivity for solid organ damage.

*IVU*

- Limited to unstable patients on their way to theatre or during surgery.
- Control then immediate and 10-minute films following 100ml of IV
  contrast medium.

*Findings*

- Is there a contralateral functioning kidney (if nephrectomy is
  considered), and is there a ureteric injury?

## Management

- Depends on severity of injury, other injuries and the stability of the
  patient, but the aim is to treat conservatively.
- Extensive devitalized tissue, active hemorrhage or a large collecting
  system injury are indicators for intervention.
- Radiological intervention includes embolizing bleeding vessels, draining
  large collections and ureteric stenting.

**Table 8.1** American Association for the Surgery of Trauma (AAST)
Classification

| Grade | Description |
|-------|-------------|
| 1 | Contusion or subcapsular haematoma |
| 2 | Superficial laceration (<1cm, not collecting duct), perinephric haematoma |
| 3 | Deep laceration (not collecting duct) |
| 4 | Laceration into collecting duct, segmental infarcts, large subcapsular haematoma |
| 5 | Shattered/devascularized kidney, vascular pedicle/renal pelvis injury |

## Further reading

**1.** American College of Radiology (2007) *ACR Appropriateness Criteria® in Renal Trauma*,
available at http://www.acr.org/SecondaryMainMenuCAtegories/quality_safety/app_criteria/pdf/
ExpertPanelonUrologic.

**2.** *Kawashima A, Sandler CM, Corl FM (2001)* Imaging of renal trauma: a comprehensive review.
*Radiographics* 2001; **21**; 557–74.

# ! ? **Renal colic**

### Definition and aetiology

Pain caused by the passage of a renal calculus through the ureter.
The most common causes of kidney stones are hypercalciuria, hyperurico-suria, hyperoxaluria, hypocitraturia, and low urinary volume.

### Epidemiology

Peak onset of symptoms aged 30–60yrs, male to female ratio of 3:1. Renal calculi affect 3% of the UK population and is increasing.

### Clinical features

Renal colic: severe, spasmodic flank pain radiating to groin/perineum.
Classically the patient is unable to lie still (in contrast to peritonitis) and has an unremarkable abdominal examination. If pyrexial, consider an infected, obstructed system and if over 60yrs look for an aortic aneurysm since the clinical presentations are similar.

### Imaging

The role of imaging is to confirm urolithiasis, identify the location and degree of obstruction, and identify potential complications. CT is probably the modality of choice due to its high sensitivity and specificity (97% and 96% respectively), although there maybe a local policy as to which to use.

#### Plain films

- Low sensitivity and specificity (45% and 75%) for urolithiasis limits its role in the acute setting.
- Can provide a baseline for follow-up.

#### Intravenous urography (IVU)

Traditionally the first-line imaging modality. Not ideal if there is poor renal function.

##### Protocol

- Control.
- Following 100ml IV contrast a 5- and 20-minute film are taken. There will be local variation in timing and delayed films may be necessary.

##### Findings

- Direct visualization of a ureteric calculus.
- A delayed nephrogram and filling of the collecting system, with a standing column of contrast in the ureter to the level of the calculus which persists post micturition.
- The length of delay in the appearance of contrast in the collecting system gives an idea of the degree of obstruction.

#### Unenhanced CT

##### Protocol

- No IV or oral contrast; full bladder; scanning prone may help differentiate between bladder and vesico-ureteric junction (VUJ) calculi and some institutions will do this routinely.
- Thin slices (<3mm) to improve detection and to facilitate multiplanar reformats.

*Findings*
- Record the number, size and position of the calculi.
- Direct signs: hydronephrosis/hydroureter down to the level of a ureteric calculus.
- Indirect signs: perinephric stranding and nephromegaly.
- Direct or indirect signs without a calculus may mean it is not visible or has recently passed. Alternatively, other causes should be considered e.g. stricture or malignancy.
- *Tissue rim sign*: a thin rim of ureter around a distal calculus helps differentiate it from a phlebolith.
- Approximately half will be negative, a third of which may have an alternative diagnosis on the scan—see Differential diagnosis.

### Ultrasound
*Protocol*
- Used mainly in pregnant and young women.
- Curvilinear probe: 3–5Mhz.
- Full bladder.

*Findings*
- Sensitive for large (>5mm) renal calculi and hydronephrosis.
- Poor for ureteric calculi unless at the VUJ.
- Useful in identifying other pathology.

## Differential diagnosis
- Aortic aneurysm
- Appendicitis, cholecystitis, diverticulitis, pancreatitis, inflammatory bowel disease, urinary tract infection (UTI)
- Ureteric malignancy
- Epididymo-orchitis, testicular torsion
- Ovarian pathology, ectopic pregnancy
- Mechanical back pain, herpes zoster

## Management
- The majority of calculi pass spontaneously with analgesia, the probability of this depends on size; 90% of 4mm, 50% of 4–7mm, and rarely if over 7mm.
- If there are signs of infection an urgent nephrostomy/ureteric stent should be considered.
- Intervention includes lithotripsy, ante/retrograde ureteric stents (to relieve obstruction), ureteroscopy and rarely surgery.

## Further reading
**1.** Tamm EP, Silverman PM and Shuman WP (2003) Evaluation of the patient with flank pain and possible ureteral calculus. *Radiology* **228**; 319–29.

**2.** Colistro R, Torreggiani WC, Lyburn ID *et al.* (2002) Unenhanced helical CT in the investigation of acute flank pain. *Clin Rad* 2002; **57**; 435–41.

**3.** Rucker CM, Menias CO and Bhaila S (2004) Mimics of renal colic: alternative diagnoses at unenhanced helical CT. *Radiographics* **24**; S11–28.

# ① ⑦ Renal obstruction

### Definition and aetiology

Although there are varying degrees of obstruction, what follows assumes that there is dilation of the collecting system (hydronephrosis) and the ureter (hydroureter). The degree of dilation depends on duration of obstruction and rate of urine production.

The more common causes are:

- *Intraluminal:* calculus, clot, transitional cell carcinoma (TCC), sloughed papilla.
- *Mural:* strictures (congenital/acquired), neuromuscular dysfunction, infection.
- *Extraluminal:* abdominal or pelvic mass/tumour, retroperitoneal fibrosis.

### Epidemiology

- *Female:* mainly gynaecological cancers and pregnancy; young (20–60yrs).
- *Males:* mainly prostatic (benign or malignant) so mostly older (>60yrs).

### Clinical features

*Acute:* flank pain, nausea and vomiting, UTI, haematuria.
*Chronic:* mostly asymptomatic; incidental finding or detected following investigation of renal failure.

### Imaging

Ultrasound is the first-line investigation. Indications for out of hours scans are the same as those for a nephrostomy, i.e. possibly infected system, solitary kidney or renal transplant.

#### Ultrasound

- Hydronephrosis progresses in the following order: dilated pelvis, dilated calices, cortex thinning.
- Hydroureter and/or bladder distention (post micturition) can indicate level of obstruction.
- Cause may be identified: calculi or tumour.
- Can take 24hrs before hydronephrosis is detectable on US.
- Raised resistive index of renal arcuate artery is an early finding.
- There may be a lack of ureteric jets on colour Doppler if obstructed.

#### IVU

- Not commonly used for diagnosing obstruction, but obstruction may be discovered on an IVU.
- In acute obstruction, dilation is an inconsistent finding.
- Obstructive nephrogram: increasingly dense for up to 3–5hrs.
- Delayed excretion of contrast may demonstrate the level of obstruction.

#### CT

Most useful for extrinsic causes.

*Protocol*
- Unenhanced imaging should be performed unless calculi are not suspected.
- A delayed excretory phase study is not always necessary as a hydroureter down to the level of obstruction can usually be seen.

*Findings*
- Signs of obstruction: hydroureter, hydronephrosis, enlarged kidney and perinephric stranding. Long-standing obstruction will result in cortical thinning.
- Cause: hydroureter to the level of obstruction. Most useful for calculus or an extrinsic mass.
- Signs of infection: poor corticomedullary differentiation, wedge-shaped areas of decreased attenuation, perinephric stranding and thickening of Gerota's fascia. Look for gas in the collecting system and parenchyma suggestive of emphysematous pyelonephritis.

## Differential diagnosis
- Non-obstructive dilation due to reflux or megacalices/ureter.

## Management
- Urgent attention is required if there are any features of infection or if there is bilateral (unilateral with a solitary kidney) hydronephrosis.
- Specific treatment depends on cause. Retrograde ureteric stents or nephrostomy +/– stents to relieve obstruction (see 📖 p. 376).
- Associated renal failure may require dialysis.

## Further reading
**1.** Georgiades CS, Moore CJ and Smith DP (2001) Differences of renal parenchymal attenuation for acutely obstructed and unobstructed kidneys on unenhanced helical CT: a useful secondary sign? *AJR* **76(4)**; 965–8.

# ⊙ Renal vein thrombosis

### Definition and aetiology

Thrombus in the renal vein due to:
- Hypercoagulable state:
  - Nephrotic syndrome
  - SLE
  - Inherited: sickle cell disease; activated protein C (APC) resistance; protein C and S deficiency; antithrombin III deficiency
- Mechanical: trauma, tumour, abscess, haematoma, aneurysm
- Dehydration: mostly in children
- Other venous thrombosis: IVC or left gonadal vein

### Epidemiology

No accurate figures since most are asymptomatic.

### Clinical features

- *Acute:* gross haematuria/proteinuria, painful flank mass, renal failure.
- *Chronic:* almost all asymptomatic. May present with renal failure or PE/DVT.

### Imaging

Doppler US is used as the initial investigation but if indeterminate, MR (if renal function impaired) or CT can be used. The findings in acute thrombosis are described below. Long-standing thrombosis leads to renal atrophy.

#### Ultrasound
- Enlarged (oedematous) kidney with hyperechoic areas (haemorrhage), loss of corticomedullary differentiation.
- Thrombus within distended renal vein.

#### CT
- Enlarged kidney, renal sinus and perinephric space oedema and coarse striations.
- Thrombus in a distended, thick-walled renal vein.

#### MRI
- Enlarged high T2 signal kidney.
- Thrombus in renal vein.

#### Venography
- Gold standard but rarely necessary due to cross-sectional imaging.
- Selective renal venography may be necessary if normal flow.

### Differential diagnosis

- Renal colic and any other cause of loin pain. Tumour can mimic thrombus but may demonstrate enhancement (CT) or internal flow (US).

## Management
- Treat the cause and anticoagulate with heparin then warfarin.
- Thrombolysis (systemic or locally) is controversial and reserved for bilateral clots, acute renal failure and failure of anticoagulation.

**Further reading**
1. Asghar M, Ahmed K, Shah SSD *et al.* (2007) Renal veint thrombosis. *Eur J Vasc Endovasc Surg* **34(2)**; 217–23.

# ① ⑦ Acute pyelonephritis

### Definition and aetiology

Inflammation of the renal parenchyma, calyces and pelvis. The majority are due to ascending infection (*E. coli*) with haematological spread (Gram +ve cocci) being less frequent.
Risk factors:

- Children: vesicoureteric reflux
- Adults: urinary obstruction, stasis and calculi.

### Epidemiology

Most common in women aged 15–30yrs.

### Clinical features

Flank pain; fever/chills; lower urinary tract symptoms (frequency, dysuria); leukocytosis; positive urine cultures.

### Imaging

Not routinely indicated in uncomplicated cases or low-risk groups.
Indications: atypical presentation, poor response or worsening on treatment, atypical organism, calculi, neuropathic bladder, immunocompromised and diabetes. All modalities may show general enlargement or focal swelling.

#### Ultrasound

- Scan *whole* abdomen (looking for other causes) with curvilinear probe (4Mhz).
- Not sensitive for diagnosis. Used to determine cause and complications.

*Findings*

- Ill defined, decreased echogenicity which is either generalized or focal.
- Calculi and/or hydronephrosis.
- The presence of gas in the collecting system suggests emphysematous pyelonephritis, (see below).
- Look for perinephric collections.

#### CT

*Protocol*

- Unenhanced if calculus suspected.
- Contrast enhanced in a portal phase (60s).

*Findings*

- With enhancement: poor corticomedullary differentiation, wedge-shaped areas of decreased attenuation, striated nephrogram
- Perinephric stranding and thickening of Gerota's fascia.
- Look for gas in the collecting system and parenchyma

#### IVU

- May demonstrate ureteric obstruction +/– calculus, although excretion decreases with severity. Now rarely used.

## Complications
- Emphysematous pyelitis (gas in pelvis and calyces) and emphysematous pyelonephritis (parenchyma, potentially fatal); associated with DM and immunocompromise.
- Perinephric or renal abscess.
- Renal scarring mainly in infants associated with vesicoureteric reflux.

## Management
- Medical: antibiotics, analgesia and hydration.
- Surgical: draining obstructed system or abscesses.

## Further reading
**1.** Craig WD, Wagner BJ and Travis MD (2008) From the archives of the AFIP: pyelonephritis: radiologic–pathologic review. *Radiographics* **28**; 255–76.

# ! ? **Epididymo-orchitis**

### Definition and aetiology

Inflammation of the epididymis and/or testicle. This is usually due to retrograde bacterial infection.

- Bacterial:
  - Prepubertal: *E. coli*, may have underlying genitourinary (GU) abnormality
  - Sexually active: chlamydia and gonorrhoea
  - Older men: *E. coli* and *Pseudomonas*, associated with outflow obstruction
- Other:
  - Chemical (reflux sterile urine), post-infectious inflammatory reaction, amiodarone, TB, brucellosis, schistosomiasis

### Epidemiology

Peak incidence 19–40yrs.

### Clinical features

Painful, erythematous and swollen epididymis/hemiscrotum. Urinary symptoms and positive urine dipstick and culture. Fever and constitutional symptoms.

*Prehn sign*: scrotal elevation decreases pain in epididymitis and not in torsion (not reliable).

### Imaging

The majority of cases are diagnosed clinically. If any imaging is required US is normally sufficient.

#### Ultrasound

*Protocol*

- High frequency linear probe (12–15MHz) appropriate to the size of patient, set on testicle/small parts.
- Be gentle, look at normal side first.

*Findings*

- Thickened epididymis which is hypo- or hyper-echoic.
- 20–40% have testicular involvement—enlarged and heterogeneous. This is non-specific but is the most common cause of the appearance. Also occurs with tumours, metastases, and infarction: *therefore should always be followed up to demonstrate complete resolution.*
- Reactive hydrocoele and scrotal wall thickening.
- Increased blood flow in the epididymis on Doppler US. Check testicular blood flow as the epididymis can become thickened in testicular torsion.
- In prepubertal patients, look for an associated underlying cause of a urinary tract infection.
- In older patients, look for evidence of bladder outflow obstruction.

## Management
- Urgent urological opinion regarding torsion in younger patients.
- Appropriate antibiotic therapy—may require a long course.
- Analgesia and scrotal support.

## Further reading
1. Dogra VS, Gottleib RH, Oka M et al. (2003) Sonography of the screen. Radiology 227; 18–36.

# ⚠ Testicular torsion

## Definition and aetiology
Rotation of the testis along the longitudinal axis of the spermatic cord.

## Epidemiology
- Most common scrotal disorder in childhood.
- Two peaks: newborns and at puberty.
- 10-fold increased risk in undescended testicle.

## Clinical features
Sudden onset of scrotal pain, often at night. Maybe associated with nausea, vomiting, scrotal swelling and tenderness, and fever.

Almost all have negative urinalysis and some have raised inflammatory markers.

The majority of diagnoses are made on clinical grounds because rapid treatment (surgery) is essential. The testicular salvage rate depends on time from onset of symptoms to surgery.

| Interval (hrs) | Salvage rate (%) |
|---|---|
| <6 | 80–100 |
| 6–12 | 75 |
| 12–24 | 20 |
| >24 | 0 |

## Imaging
Imaging of testicular torsion is controversial as it can never be excluded. Surgery should never be delayed in order to confirm the diagnosis. The two options are described below, although only ultrasound is in common use due to speed and availability (particularly out of hours).

### Ultrasound
*Protocol*
- High-frequency linear probe, appropriate to the size of patient, used with testicle/small parts settings.
- If the clinician is unable to examine the scrotum, the likelihood of a diagnostic ultrasound is low.

*Findings*
- Absent testicular and epididymal flow on colour duplex is the only specific finding. **The presence of flow does not exclude torsion.**
- Non-specific findings include: swollen and hypoechoic testicle and epididymis, thickened spermatic cord, thickened scrotal wall and occasionally a hydrocoele.

### MRI
*Protocol*
- T2-weighted, T2*-weighted, and dynamic contrast enhancement (DCE). T1 weighted.

*Findings*
- Normal or enlarged testicle with heterogeneous, low T2 signal.
- Decreased or no perfusion on DCE.
- Whirlpool appearance of the cord.

## Differential diagnosis
- Epididymo-orchitis
- Scrotal abscess
- Torsion of testicular or epididymal appendage
- Trauma
- Testicular tumour

## Management
- Urgent surgery: detorting the effected side and bilateral orchidopex

## Further reading
**1.** Aso C, Enriquex G, Fité M *et al.* (2005) Gray-scale and color Doppler sonography of scrotal disorders in children: an update. *Radiographics* **25**; 1197–214. (DOI: 10.1148/rg.255045109.)

# ☼ ① Testicular trauma

### Definition and aetiology

Trauma can result in contusion, haematoma, haematocoele, rupture/fracture or dislocation of the testis (see below for description). It is caused by:
- *Blunt*: 85%; sporting injury, assault/kick, RTA, falls and straddle injury.
- *Penetrating*: 15%; stab and gunshot wounds, and animal bites.
- *Degloving* (scrotal): rare; machinery injury.

Testicular rupture: tear in the tunica albuginea (fibrous connective tissue surround testis) resulting in extrusion of the testicular contents.

### Epidemiology

Despite their exposed location, trauma is uncommon. Mostly seen in the 10–30 year age range.

### Clinical features

Most injuries are unilateral and isolated. They usually present early with pain, nausea and vomiting. Scrotal swelling and bruising raises the suspicion of significant injury.

### Imaging

Most penetrating injuries and clinically obvious testis ruptures will undergo immediate surgical exploration. The main role of imaging is to look for less obvious rupture as this is a surgical emergency with an 80% salvage rate if operated on within 72hrs.

#### Ultrasound

*Protocol*

High-frequency linear probe on testicle/small parts setting.
Press gently after adequate analgesia.

*Findings*
- *Rupture*: interruption of tunica albuginea (rarely seen; <20%), heterogeneous testis (haemorrhage/infarction) with irregular border (most consistent finding), scrotal wall thickening, and a large haematocoele.
- *Fracture*: linear hypoechoic band extending across the parenchyma but overall smooth contour and shape remain. If vascular integrity is seen on Doppler US, then this can be managed conservatively.
- *Haematocoele*: blood collection within the tunica vaginalis (serous membrane pouch surrounding the testis); up to 80% are associated with fracture. They have an appearance similar to a hydrocoele but are complex and hyperechoic. They may be due to extra- or intratesticular bleeding, abnormal testicular parenchyma suggest rupture of the haematocoele.
- *Haematoma*: of the testis, epididymis, or scrotal wall. Acute blood appears hyperechoic but becomes complex with cystic components with time.
- *Dislocation*: testis dislocated secondary to blunt trauma. Uncommon (0.5% of abdominal trauma), mostly due to motorcycle accidents and 1/3 are bilateral. New locations include: superficial, inguinal, pubic, penile, intra-abdominal, retrovesical, perineal, and crural. *On a CT performed for trauma always check the scrotum; it may not have been detected clinically.*

- Doppler blood flow to the testis indicates an intact vascular pedicle. Absence of flow implies a torsion or spermatic cord injury.
- 10–15% of tumours present after trauma. If surgery is not undertaken, *all testicular abnormalities require follow-up.*

*MRI*
- Described in the literature as useful in equivocal cases but not routinely used.
- May be helpful in locating dislocated testis.

**Differential diagnosis**
- Pelvic/abdominal trauma
- Epididyo-orchitis
- Testicular tumour

**Management**
- Indications for exploration:
  - Clinical findings consistent with testicular injury; expanding or large haematocoeles (>5cm); dislocation refractory to manual reduction; penetrating or degloving injuries. Smaller collections may be evacuated for pain relief.
  - US: disruption of the tunica albuginea or absence of blood flow.
- Surgery is performed for debridement, irrigation, haemostasis and closue of the tunica albuginea.
- Conservative management includes analgesia, NSAIDs, bed rest, support and ice packs.

**Further reading**

1. Deurdulian C, Mittelstaedt CA, Chiong WK *et al.* (2007) US of acute scrotal trauma: optimal technique, imaging findings, and management. *RadioGraphics* **27**; 357–69.

2. Dogra VS, Gottleib RH, Oka M *et al.* Sonography of the scrotum. *Radiology* **227**; 18–36.

3. Buckley JC and McAninch JW (2006) Use of ultrasonography for the diagnosis of testicular injuries in blunt scrotal trauma. *J Urol* **175(1)**; 175–8.

# ☼ ⊕ ① Urethral injury

### Definition and aetiology

*Anterior* (penile and bulbar): blunt perineal injury; straddle or kicked; can present late.

*Posterior* (membranous and prostatic): most due to RTA/falls with associated pelvic fractures (10%).

*Iatrogenic injuries* (catheterization): can affect the whole length.

### Clinical features

Haematuria, urinary retention, blood at the urethral meatus and a high riding prostate on rectal examination.

### Imaging

#### Retrograde urethrogram

*Protocol*

Using aseptic technique a 16–18 Fr Foley catheter is inserted approximately 2cm and the balloon inflated within the navicular fossa (1–2ml air). A control image is taken and then continuous screening is performed while gently injecting water-soluble contrast (e.g. Urografin®).

*Findings*

- Normal: outline full length of urethra with bladder filling. The catheter can then be advanced into the bladder if required.
- Stretching of the urethra produces a narrowing and elevation of the bladder due to haematoma.
- Anterior tears show extravasation into the perineum, and posterior ones into the retropubic space.
- In partial tears there is filling of the bladder.

#### CT

Not performed specifically for urethral injury but imaging findings on a CT scan performed for trauma suggestive of urethral injury (especially if there is a pelvic fracture) are:

- Prostatic elevation, urine/contrast extravasation, distortion or obscuration of the urogenital diaphragm fat plane, and haematoma of the ischiocavernosus/bulbocavernosus/obturator internus muscles.

### Differential diagnosis

- Traumatic haematuria: bladder, ureter or renal injury

### Management

- Surgery for complete tears
- Conservative management with catheterisation for partial tears

### Further reading

**1.** Ali M, Safriel Y, Sclafani JA et al. (2003) CT signs of urethral injury. *Radiographics* **23**; 951–63.

**2.** Kawashima A, Sandler CM, Wasserman NF et al. (2004) Imaging of urethral disease: a pictorial review. *Radiographics* **24**; S195–216.

# Central nervous system

Daniel Scoffings

# ☣ ⊙ **Acute ischaemic stroke**

### Definition
'Stroke' is a clinical syndrome in which there is rapid onset of focal or global neurological signs which are of presumed vascular origin and which lasts at least 24hrs.

### Aetiology
85% of strokes are ischaemic and 15% are haemorrhagic. Clinical history and examination cannot differentiate between these causes, for which imaging is necessary. Causes of ischaemic stroke include large vessel atherosclerosis, cardioembolism and small vessel disease.

### Clinical features
These depend on which areas of the brain undergo infarction. Unilateral weakness, numbness, visual field defects and dysphasia are the most common.

### Imaging
The key feature is that abnormalities correspond to arterial territories (Fig. 9.1). Large vessel infarcts involve both the cortex and the underlying white matter.

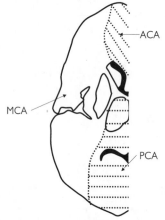

**Fig 9.1** Cerebral vascular territories at level of basal ganglia.
ACA, MCA, PCA: anterior, middle and posterior cerebral arteries.

## CT

High sensitivity for haemorrhage, widespread availability and ease of access mean that unenhanced CT remains the first line imaging technique in the UK.

- Review images on 'stroke windows' (WL 32 HU, WW 8 HU) in addition to conventional settings (WL 40 HU, WW 80 HU) to increase sensitivity for early ischaemic oedema.
- Look for haemorrhage (attenuation of clotted blood is 45–75 HU, but can be lower in anaemia).
- Look for hyperattenuating artery sign:
  - Unilateral increased density of artery—distal internal carotid artery (ICA), trunk or branches of middle cerebral artery (MCA), basilar artery (BA), proximal posterior cerebral artery (PCA), specific for occlusion but relatively insensitive.
  - Mimicked by calcification and increased haematocrit, but these cause hyperattenuation of all intracranial vessels.
- Evaluate for early ischaemic oedema:
  - Obscuration of lentiform nucleus.
  - Loss of insular ribbon (i.e. low attenuation in insular cortex and subjacent white matter).
  - Loss of grey–white interface in arterial distribution.
  - Reduced attenuation of >1/3 of MCA territory (contraindication to thrombolysis).
- Swelling of ischaemic brain:
  - Sulcal effacement.
  - Ventricular compression.
- Low attenuation of cortex and underlying white matter in arterial territory distribution.

## MRI

### Protocol

Axial T2W, FLAIR, gradient echo, diffusion-weighted imaging (DWI), MRA of intracranial and neck vessels.

### Findings

- T2W/FLAIR (fluid-attenuated inversion recovery): increased signal in cortex and underlying white matter.
- Gradient echo: low signal in areas of haemorrhage.
- DWI: restricted diffusion in acute infarcts (<10 days) appears as high signal on DWI and low signal on the map of apparent diffusion coefficient (ADC).
- MRA: vascular occlusion or stenosis.

## Differential diagnosis

- Encephalitis and low-grade gliomas can resemble acute infarcts but do not conform to vascular territories. Low-grade gliomas typically have a slightly rounded margin in contrast to the wedge shape of an infarct. Subacute infarcts and tumours can both enhance after IV contrast medium but infarcts classically show a gyriform pattern of enhancement. The sudden onset of symptoms distinguishes an infarct from the more subacute presentation of encephalitis and tumour.

## Complications
- Haemorrhagic transformation: occurs in 20–40% within 1 week of ictus, may be asymptomatic, petechial haemorrhage or space-occupying and associated with clinical deterioration.
- 'Malignant' MCA infarction: severe ischaemic oedema and swelling resulting in raised intracranial pressure and brain shift. Fatal in 80%.

## Treatment
Intravenous thrombolysis with tissue plasminogen activator reduces morbidity and mortality if given within 3hrs of onset. Intra-arterial thrombolysis is effective up to 6hrs after onset. Contraindications include:
- Intracranial haemorrhage.
- Involvement of more than 1/3 of the MCA territory on the initial CT.
- Seizure at stroke onset.
- Prior stroke in the last 3 months.
- Heparin treatment in last 48hrs and thromboplastin time above upper limit of normal.
- Thrombocytopaenia (platelets <100 000/mm$^3$).
- Systolic BP >185 mmHg or diastolic >110 mmHg.
- Blood glucose <2.8mmol/L or >22mmol/L.

## Further reading
**1.** Srinivasan A, Goyal M, Al Azri F et al. (2006) State of the art imaging of acute stroke. *RadioGraphics* **26**; S75–S95.

# ⚠ **Cerebral venous sinus thrombosis**

### Aetiology

A predisposing cause can be found in 80%. Commonest risk factors are pregnancy, oral contraceptive use, dehydration, infection (sinusitis, mastoiditis), trauma and sinus compression by tumour.

### Clinical features

Presentation is subacute in 50%, acute in 30% and chronic in 20%.
Headache is the commonest feature; papilloedema, seizures and focal neurological deficits also occur.

### Imaging

#### CT

*Findings*

- Increased attenuation (approx. 45–75 HU) in thrombosed sinus (seen in 20–50%) or internal cerebral veins.
  - Sinuses also appear dense in dehydration and with an elevated haematocrit.
  - Compare sinuses with arteries to check for generalized increase in attenuation unrelated to thrombosis.
- Sulcal effacement and brain swelling.
- Low attenuation oedema/venous infarction:
  - Does not correspond to an arterial territory.
  - Bilateral thalamic low attenuation with thrombosis of deep cerebral venous system.
- Subcortical haemorrhage.
- With IV contrast may see 'empty delta' (Fig. 9.2) of enhancing dura around thrombus in superior sagittal sinus (in 25–75%).

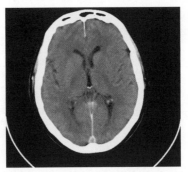

**Fig 9.2** Empty delta sign.

### CT venography
*Protocol*
- Volume acquisition from C1 to vertex (1mm collimation).
- 100ml of 300mg I/ml contrast at 2ml/sec.
- Start scanning at 45s.

*Findings*
- Review source images, 2D MPR and 2D MIP (WL 130 HU, WW 260 HU).
- Look for thrombus as a non-enhancing filling defect.
- Dilated transmedullary venous collaterals may be seen.

### MRI
- MRI more sensitive than CT to the parenchymal sequelae of venous thrombosis (seen in 57%).

*Findings*
- Loss of sinus flow void.
- Compare signal intensity in two orthogonal planes to exclude flow effects.
- Signal of thrombus varies with its age:

|      | Normal           | Acute (<5d) | Subacute (6–15d) | Chronic (>15d) |
|------|------------------|-------------|------------------|----------------|
| T1W  | Variable         | Isointense  | High             | Iso/high       |
| T2W  | Low (flow void)  | Low         | High             | Iso/high       |

- Focal oedema (25%): high signal on T2W; low signal on T1W.
- Haemorrhage (32%): variable signal.
- Variable appearances on DWI:
  - Cytotoxic oedema: high signal on DWI, low on apparent diffusion coefficient (ADC) map, affects cortex mainly.
  - Vasogenic oedema: low signal on DWI, high on ADC map, tends to be restricted to white matter.
- Distribution of parenchymal changes varies with site of thrombosis:
  - Bilateral parasagittal → superior sagittal sinus.
  - Temporal lobe → transverse sinus.
  - Bilateral thalami, basal ganglia → deep venous system/straight sinus.

### MR venography
*Protocol*
- 2D time of flight (2D–TOF), 3D phase contrast (3D–PC) or contrast-enhanced MRV.

*Findings*
- Thrombus appears as flow gaps or filling defects in the affected sinus.
- Correlate with appearance on T1W and T2W to confirm thrombus and exclude flow effects.

- Subacute thrombus has high signal on T1W and can 'shine through' on TOF MRV and give false impression of normal flow.

**Differential diagnosis**

- Sinuses appear dense on CT in patients with polycythaemia
- Focal filling defects from arachnoid granulations (superior sagittal sinus > transverse sinus)
- Hypoplasia/atresia of transverse sinus (20%, usually left-sided)
- Idiopathic intracranial hypertension (flow gaps in anterior aspects of transverse sinuses caused by extrinsic compression)

**Treatment**

Management includes treatment of the underlying/predisposing condition (e.g. antibiotics for sinusitis), systemic anticoagulation, treatment of raised intracranial pressure and symptomatic treatment (e.g. anticonvulsants). In refractory cases, local thrombolysis and interventional techniques aimed at mechanical disruption/aspiration of the thrombus may be attempted.

**Further reading**

**1.** Leach JL, Fortuna RB, Jones BV et al. (2006) Imaging of cerebral venous thrombosis: current techniques, spectrum of findings, and diagnostic pitfalls. *Radiographics* **26**; S5–18.

**2.** Rodallec MH, Krainik A, Feydy A et al. (2006) Cerebral venous thrombosis and multidetector CT angiography: tips and tricks. *RadioGraphics* **26**; S19–41.

# ① Subarachnoid haemorrhage

## Aetiology

Aneurysm rupture is the most common cause of spontaneous SAH. Other causes include AVMs, dural AV fistulas, cerebral venous sinus thrombosis, intracranial arterial dissection and spinal vascular malformations. Non-aneurysmal perimesencephalic haemorrhage, which accounts for 15–20%, is thought to have a venous cause.

## Clinical features

Sudden onset of severe headache is typical. Focal neurological deficits or reduced GCS may be present. Neck stiffness and photophobia may take several hours to develop.

## Imaging

### CT

- Unenhanced CT is the most sensitive imaging investigation.
- Sensitivity for SAH decreases with time from ictus:
  - 98% in first 12hrs
  - 93% at 24hrs
  - 80% at 5 days
  - 50% after 7 days

*Findings*

- Look for increased attenuation in cortical sulci, Sylvian fissures, interhemispheric fissure and basal cisterns (Fig. 9.3)
- If no SAH seen, check review areas:
  - Interpeduncular cistern
  - Suprasellar cistern
  - Occipital horns of lateral ventricles, posterior third ventricle and fourth ventricle
  - Foramen magnum
- Look for complications:
  - Hydrocephalus (obstructive or communicating)
  - Parenchymal ischaemia due to vasospasm (peaks at 4–7 days)

⚠ A negative CT does not exclude SAH. Even if scanned immediately, 2% of patients will have a negative CT and the percentage increases rapidly after this. Patients in whom SAH is suspected but who have a negative CT should undergo lumbar puncture no sooner than 12hrs after ictus to look for CSF xanthochromia.

### CT angiography

*Protocol*

Exact protocols vary with the machine used. For example:

- MDCT: e.g. 16 slice × 0.75mm collimation. Pitch 0.85.
- 100ml of 300mg I/ml contrast injected at 5 ml/s.
- Imaging triggered from a bolus track in the aortic arch.
- Image from C1–2 to vertex.

*Findings*

- Review source images first as these will contain information that may be lost with later MIP and volume-rendered reconstructions.

- Scrutinize common sites of aneurysms:
  - Anterior communicating artery
  - Posterior communicating artery
  - MCA bifurcation
  - Basilar tip
  - Posterior inferior cerebellar arteries.
- Distribution of blood on initial CT may point to likely source, but can be unreliable.

### Differential diagnosis

- Pseudosubarachnoid haemorrhage: relative increased attenuation of vessels in basal cisterns and Sylvian fissures caused by diffuse cerebral oedema reducing the attenuation of adjacent brain.

### Complications

- Hydrocephalus
- Intraventricular/intracerebral extension of haemorrhage
- Vasospasm and cerebral ischaemia

### Treatment

Initial management includes supportive measures such as analgesia and antiemetics. Nimodipine reduces the risk of delayed ischaemic deficits. External ventricular drainage may be needed to treat hydrocephalus. Definitive management of a ruptured aneurysm may be endovascular occlusion with detachable platinum coils or neurosurgical clipping.

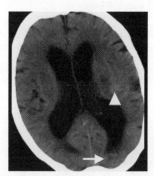

**Fig 9.3** Subarachnoid haemorrhage in Sylvian fissure (arrowhead) and haemorrhage in occipital horn of lateral ventricle (arrow).

### Further reading

**1.** Goddard AJP, Tan G and Becker J (2005) Computed tomography angiography: for the detection and characterization of intra-cranial aneurysms: current status.*Clin Radiol* **60**; 1221–36.

**2.** Al-Shahi R, White PM, Davenport RJ *et al.* (2006) Subarachnoid haemorrhage. *BMJ* **333**; 235–40.

# ① Intracerebral haemorrhage

## Aetiology

- Cerebral amyloid angiopathy 40–60%.
- Hypertension 15%.
- Vascular malformation 15–25%.
- Other causes: vasculitis, venous thrombosis, haemorrhagic transformation of arterial infarcts, illicit drugs, e.g. cocaine and amphetamine, tumours.

## Clinical features

Patients may present with headache, vomiting, seizures, coma or focal neurological deficits.

## Imaging: general features

### CT

- Acute haematoma appears as a well-defined area of increased attenuation (approx. 45–75 HU).
- Surrounding low attenuation rim initially due to clot retraction and extrusion of serum, later on perihaematomal vasogenic oedema develops.
- Haematoma can enlarge in first 24hrs and may be associated with clinical deterioration.
- Progressive decrease in attenuation from periphery inwards with resolution, resulting in ill-defined margins in subacute stage.
- Slit-like low attenuation, or area of cerebromalacia (low attenuation and volume loss) in chronic stage.

### MRI

- Signal changes in haematoma are complex and depend on oxygenation of haemoglobin, local environment of haematoma, and magnetic field strength as well as other factors.
- Signal changes progress from periphery to centre of haematoma with haemoglobin in different oxygenation states within the same lesion.

|  | State of Hb | T1W | T2W |
|---|---|---|---|
| Hyperacute (<few hrs) | Oxy-Hb | Iso/low | High |
| Acute (hrs–days) | Deoxy-Hb | Iso/low | Low |
| Early subacute (first few days) | Met-Hb (intracellular) | High | Low |
| Late subacute (days–months) | Met-Hb (extracellular) | High | High |
| Chronic (months–years) | Haemosiderin | Iso/low | Low |

### Hypertensive haemorrhage

- Typical locations include lentiform nucleus (65%), thalamus (20%), pons (10%) and cerebellum (5%).

*Cerebral amyloid angiopathy*
- Typically occurs in older, normotensive patients.
- Haemorrhage in a cortical–subcortical location is characteristic.
- Borders of the haemorrhage are often irregular.
- Any lobe can be involved. The deep white matter, basal ganglia and brainstem are spared.
- May be associated with SAH, Subdural haemorrhage (SDH) or intraventricular haemorrhage.
- Associated with a leukoencephalopathy (low attenuation on CT, high signal on T2W MRI).
- Multiple microhaemorrhages (<5mm) in cortical–subcortical location are best shown by T2*W gradient echo MRI because of 'blooming' artefact.

*Tumours*
Tumours with propensity for haemorrhage can be primary (glioblastoma, oligodendroglioma, primitive neuroectodermal tumour) or secondary (melanoma, renal cell, thyroid, choriocarcinoma). It is often not possible to determine that an acute haemorrhage is due to underlying tumour, and follow-up imaging is often necessary. This may show:
- Presence of enhancing tissue that is not haematoma.
- Delayed evolution of blood products and an irregular or incomplete ring of haemosiderin at MRI.
- Persistent oedema and mass effect beyond that expected for a 'benign' haematoma.

*Vascular malformations*
- Suggestive features of an AVM include foci of calcification in the nidus, and abnormal feeding/draining vessels, which appear as serpentine areas of enhancement on CT and as flow voids on MRI.
- Cavernous malformations typically have a 'popcorn' appearance of heterogeneous signal, reflecting blood degradation products of varying ages. Lesions can be multiple in up to 25% and are best detected with T2*W MRI.

## Complications
Mass effect may cause brain herniation and hydrocephalus.

## Treatment
Haematomas that exert significant mass effect, particularly in the posterior fossa, may require surgical evacuation. In most instances, treatment is supportive.

## Further reading
**1.** Chao CP, Kotsenas AL and Broderick DF (2006) Cerebral amyloid angiopathy: CT and MR imaging findings. *Radiographics* **26**; 1517–31.

# ⓘ Carotid and vertebral artery dissection

### Definition

Dissection refers to intramural haemorrhage within an artery. It can be subintimal (haemorrhage between the tunica intima and media) or, less often, subadventitial (deep to the investing tunica adventitia).

### Aetiology

Most cases are preceded by trauma, which can be trivial. Spontaneous dissection also occurs. Predisposing conditions include fibromuscular dysplasia, Marfan's syndrome and Ehlers–Danlos syndrome type IV.

### Clinical features

Neck pain and headache are common (75%). Carotid dissection may cause retro-orbital headache and Horner's syndrome. Stroke occurs early with intracranial dissection but can be delayed up to several weeks with extracranial dissection. Dissection causes 20% of strokes in patients under 30 years.

### Imaging

ICA dissection most often occurs just cranial to the common carotid artery (CCA) bifurcation. Vertebral dissection is commonest at the C1–2 level. Catheter angiography is the 'gold standard' investigation but CTA and MRI are both sensitive and accurate.

#### *CT angiography*

*Protocol*

Exact protocols depend on the machine used. Coverage should extend from aortic arch to the circle of Willis.

*Findings*

Review axial source images and multiplanar MIPs. Features of dissection on CTA include:

- Narrowed lumen (centric or eccentric) surrounded by crescentic mural thickening.
- Increased arterial diameter.
- Occluded lumen (tapered or abrupt) with increased arterial diameter.
- Alternatively, the lumen may be narrowed and dilated.
- Intimal flap.

#### *MRI*

*Protocol*

Image the brain as for ischaemic stroke (📖 p. 208). Obtain axial fat-suppressed T1W images through the neck and MRA of neck vessels.

*Findings*

- Brain findings as for acute ischaemic stroke.
- Periarterial rim of intramural haematoma is key finding:
  - Usually eccentric, may be circumferential.
  - Typically widens artery.

- Signal intensity depends on time since dissection:
  - Iso/slightly hyperintense to muscle on T1W/T2W in first few days.
  - Hyperintense thereafter and remains abnormal for months.
  - May enhance.
- Focal areas of narrowing/signal loss on MRA.

## Differential diagnosis

Severe atherosclerotic stenosis may produce rim of high signal in affected vessel, but this is usually isointense to muscle on T1W.

## Treatment

There are no evidence-based guidelines for treatment. One approach is anticoagulation with heparin or low molecular weight heparin for 1–2 weeks followed by 3–6 months warfarin.

## Further reading

**1.** Elijovich L, Kazmi K, Gauvrit JY et al. (2006) The emerging role of multidetector row CT angiography in the diagnosis of cervical arterial dissection: preliminary study. *Neuroradiology* **48**; 606–12.

# ① Head injury

### Aetiology

Motor vehicle accidents account for most cases of serious head injury, other causes include falls and assault.

### Clinical features

Reduced GCS, seizure, headache, amnesia or vomiting may occur. There may be signs of a skull base fracture, such as bilateral periorbital haematoma, mastoid process bruising or cerebral spinal fluid (CSF) otorrhoea/rhinorrhoea.

### Imaging

CT is the modality of choice for evaluating acute head trauma. Images should be reviewed on standard brain windows and also reconstructed with an edge-enhancing 'bone algorithm' to be viewed on bone windows. Indications for emergency head CT imaging have been discussed (see 📖 p. 44).

#### Skull fractures

- Calvarial fractures may be hard to see, particularly if undisplaced and parallel to the plane of section.
- Petrous temporal bone fractures are longitudinal in 80%, transverse in 20%.
- Occipital condyle fractures can be classified as type I (impaction), type II (extension of basal skull fracture), and type III (avulsion). Of these, type III is regarded as unstable.
- Pneumocephalus most often occurs when a fracture involves the para-nasal sinuses or mastoid air cells, but may be seen with a calvarial fracture that extends through the skin and dura.

#### Extradural haematoma (EDH)

- A lentiform shape is typical; EDHs do not cross cranial sutures unless they are diastased. They can cross the midline, unlike subdural haematoma.
- An associated fracture is present in 90%.
- Low attenuation within the haematoma ('swirl sign') indicates active haemorrhage.
- Bleeding typically has an arterial source, often from the middle meningeal artery.

#### Subdural haematoma (SDH)

- Characteristically crescent-shaped; they can cross cranial sutures but are reflected alongside the falx when they reach the midline.
- Bleeding arises from veins that cross the subdural space. Cerebral atrophy in elderly or alcoholic patients stretches these veins and predisposes to SDH.
- Small SDH may be obscured by adjacent skull – widen the windows to assess this.

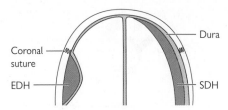

**Fig. 9.4** Extra- and subdural haematomas.

### Contusions
- Commonest in inferior frontal lobes, anterior and lateral temporal lobes.
- Low attenuation if non-haemorrhagic, increased attenuation when haemorrhage present.
- Enlargement is common in first 48hrs, may be accompanied by vasogenic oedema.
- With resolution, focal brain atrophy occurs.

### Diffuse axonal injury
- Axonal shearing injuries most often occur at cortico-medullary junction, posterior body and splenium of corpus callosum. With more severe injury, the basal ganglia and dorsolateral brainstem are involved.
- Initial CT is often normal, may see small (0.5–1.5cm) haemorrhages with surrounding oedema on delayed scans.
- MRI is the most sensitive investigation:
  - High signal on T2W
  - Low signal on T2*W gradient echo if haemorrhagic
  - High signal on DWI, low signal on ADC map (i.e. restricted diffusion).

### Brain herniation (Fig. 9.5)
- *Subfalcine herniation* causes displacement of midline structures that is more marked anteriorly. Displacement of septum pellucidum by >15 mm is associated with poor prognosis.
- *Uncal herniation* results in medial displacement of the uncus, effacement of the lateral suprasellar cistern and, in severe cases, displacement of the brainstem.
- *Descending transtentorial herniation* appears as effacement of perimesencephalic cisterns. Ascending transtentorial herniation occurs with mass effect in the posterior fossa and results in displacement of the superior vermis through the tentorial hiatus.
- *Tonsillar herniation* >5mm below the foramen magnum is abnormal but can be difficult to assess with CT. Anterior displacement of medulla and effacement of CSF at the foramen magnum distinguish herniation from normal low-lying tonsils (Fig. 9.6).

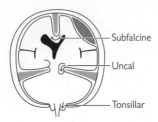

**Fig. 9.5** Brain herniations.

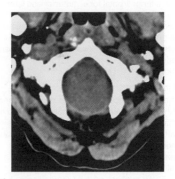

**Fig. 9.6** Tonsillar herniation.

### Treatment

Neurosurgical intervention may be required to relieve mass effect from EDH or SDH. In cases of raised intracranial pressure (ICP) that is refractory to medical management, decompressive craniectomy may be undertaken.

## Spinal cord trauma

# :☼: ① Spinal cord trauma

### Aetiology

Motor vehicle accidents, assault, falls and sports injuries are the most common causes.

### Clinical features

- *Tetraplegia* occurs with injury to cervical segments of the cord.
- *Paraplegia* results from damage to the thoracic, lumbar or sacral segments.
- *Complete* injury is one in which there is total loss of motor and sensory function three segments below the neurologically injured level.

### Imaging

#### CT

CT is the best modality for assessing the vertebrae for fractures and dislocations but is insensitive to spinal cord injury.

#### MR

*Protocol*

Sagittal and axial imaging with T1W and T2W sequences. Sagittal fat-suppressed T2W or STIR improve detection of associated ligamentous injuries. T2*W gradient echo increases sensitivity to cord haemorrhage.

*Findings*

- Haemorrhage:
  - Most often occurs in central grey matter at the level of mechanical impact.
  - Low signal on T2W and gradient echo in acute stage (deoxyHb).
  - High signal on T1W in subacute stage, which may be delayed for 8 days or more (metHb).
  - Haemorrhage >10mm long on sagittal images are suggestive of complete injury and poor prognosis.
- Oedema (non-haemorrhagic contusion):
  - High signal on T2W for variable length above/below level of impact.
  - Length correlates with degree of neurological deficit.
- Swelling:
  - Focal cord enlargement centred at level of mechanical impact.
  - Best assessed on sagittal T1W.

### Complications

- Spinal cord cyst/syrinx.
- Myelomalacia.
- Cord tethering.

### Treatment

The role of high-dose methylprednisolone is controversial. Supportive treatment is aimed at preventing cardiovascular and respiratory complications and pressure sores.

# ⑦ Intracranial tumour

## Definitions
Intra-axial tumours are those that are located within the brain parenchyma. Extra-axial tumours originate outside of the brain.

## Aetiology and epidemiology
In adults the commonest intra-axial tumours are metastases and glioblastoma multiforme. Meningioma is the most frequent extra-axial tumour.

## Clinical features
Headache, new-onset seizures, focal neurological disturbance, confusion and personality change can all occur.

## Imaging: general features
MRI is better than CT for assessing intracranial tumours. The first thing to establish is whether a tumour is intra- or extra-axial, since this directs the differential diagnosis. Findings indicative of an extra-axial lesion include:
- Rim of CSF signal between lesion and brain surface.
- Flow voids within surface vessels between lesion and brain.
- Focal widening of CSF spaces at the margins of the lesion.
- Cortex between mass and white matter.

Other findings are only suggestive of extra-axial location:
- Broad-base along inner table of skull, or on the falx cerebri.
- Changes in overlying bone.

*Metastases*
- Solitary in up to 50%.
- Most often located at grey-white matter junction. Commonest cerebellar tumour in adults.
- Enhancement is typical (lesions lack blood–brain barrier) and can be solid or ring-like.
- Usually surrounded by vasogenic oedema in white matter that is disproportionate to the size of the lesion.
- Haemorrhagic metastases: most often melanoma, renal, thyroid and choriocarcinoma.

*Low-grade glioma*
- Appear as focal area of low attenuation on CT, low signal on T1W and high signal on T2W at MRI.
- Involves white matter and may extend to cortex.
- Differentiated from cerebral infarct by lack of conformity to arterial territory and often by the presence of slightly rounded margins.
- Presence of calcification is suggestive of oligodendroglioma.
- Enhancement is usually absent.

*High-grade glioma*
- Enhancement is typical, often as an irregular and nodular ring surrounding a non-enhancing area of necrosis.
- Modest amounts of vasogenic oedema in surrounding white matter.

*Primary CNS lymphoma*
- A periventricular location is classical. Lesions abut ependyma or pia in 75%.
- Lymphoma is slightly hyperdense on CT and low signal on T2W MRI because of high nucleus-to-cytoplasm ratio.
- Homogeneous enhancement is typical in immunocompetent patients. Lymphoma in immunocompromised patients shows ring enhancement.

*Meningioma*
- Typically slightly hyperdense on CT, isointense on T1W and T2W MRI
- Calcification present in 20%
- Hyperostotic change in adjacent skull in 20%
- Vasogenic oedema in white matter of adjacent brain in up to 40%
- Homogeneous enhancement is typical
- An enhancing dural 'tail' is seen alongside the tumour in 70% and is highly suggestive of meningioma (though not pathognomonic)

## Differential diagnosis

The differential diagnosis of a ring-enhancing lesion includes high-grade glioma, metastasis and abscess.
- Abscesses tend to have a thin rim of enhancement that is thinner towards the lateral ventricles whilst tumours show more irregular and nodular enhancement. DWI is helpful in distinguishing abscesses from tumour, abscess shows restricted diffusion in its centre whilst tumours do not (if they show any restricted diffusion it is in the enhancing part).

## Treatment

Dexamethasone can be used to reduce associated oedema. Depending on tumour location, patient's symptoms and performance status, neurosurgical options include biopsy, debulking and gross resection.

Radiotherapy and chemotherapy may be offered once a histological diagnosis has been obtained.

# ① **Metastatic spinal cord compression**

## Aetiology

Breast, lung, and prostate cancer are the commonest causes. Renal cancer, lymphoma and myeloma are less frequent.

## Clinical features

Pain is the commonest presenting symptom (>90%), followed by weakness and sensory disturbance (>50%), sphincter incontinence and urinary hesitancy or retention.

## Imaging

### MR

*Protocol*

Sagittal T1W, T2W of whole spine (multilevel disease in up to 50%). Axial T1W, T2W through areas of abnormality. Adequate pain relief is essential to avoid a non-diagnostic study caused by patient motion. Fat-suppressed T2W or STIR sequences increase conspicuity of tumour in affected vertebrae, but T1W sequences alone may be sufficient to determine which levels require radiotherapy.

*Findings*

- Level of involvement is thoracic in 50–70%, lumbosacral in 20–30% and cervical in 10–30%. Site of pain and sensory level do not correlate exactly with actual level of compression in most cases.
- T1W is the most useful sequence to detect bone metastases:
  - Tumour is low signal compared to normal marrow.
  - Diffuse metastatic replacement is suspected if marrow is of lower signal than intervertebral discs.
- T2W shows tumour as high signal (prostate metastases are usually low signal).
- Collapse of vertebral body may occur, with retropulsion of bone into canal.
- Tumour extension into epidural space and neural foraminae can be hard to see on T1W, and can require T2W or post-gadolinium T1W.
- Compression diagnosed when mass displaces, indents, or causes complete loss of cord/cauda equina definition (Fig. 9.7).
- Thecal sac may be compressed without compression of the spinal cord.
- If no compression seen, consider possibility of intradural extramedullary metastases or intramedullary metastases and obtain post-gadolinium imaging:
  - Intradural extramedullary tumour most often appears as lumbosacral nodules: low signal on T1W and T2W, showing enhancement.
  - Intramedullary metastases are most often solitary, oval lesions, that do not expand the cord and are isointense on T1W, high signal on T2W. Contrast enhancement is typical.

## Treatment

Outcome is significantly better when patients are treated before neurological compromise has occurred. Delays in referral and investigation are common and result in poor outcomes.

External beam radiotherapy is the usual treatment for metastatic spinal cord compression; high-dose corticosteroids have an adjunctive role. Surgery may be considered for intractable pain where further radiotherapy cannot be given, and in cases with spinal instability.

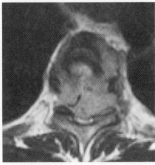

**Fig. 9.7** Metastatic spinal cord compression.

## Further reading

**1.** Adbi S, Adams CI, Foweraker KL *et al.* (2005) Metastatic spinal cord syndromes: imaging appearances and treatment planing. *Clin Radiol* **60**; 637–47.

**2.** Johnons AJ, Ying J, El Gammal T *et al.* (2007) Which MR imaging sequences are necessary in determining the need for radiation therapy for cord compression? A prospective study. *Am J Neuroradiol* **26**; 32–37.

# ⓘ **Meningitis and encephalitis**

### Definitions

Meningitis is inflammation of the meninges, and may be bacterial, viral, granulomatous, fungal or carcinomatous. Encephalitis refers to inflammation of the brain parenchyma.

# **Meningitis**

### Aetiology

The causes of bacterial meningitis vary with age; S. pneumoniae and N. meningitidis are most common in adults and children.

### Clinical features

Headache, fever, photophobia and meningism are classic features of meningitis.

### Imaging

#### CT

⚠ CT is often requested to determine if it is safe to perform a lumbar puncture (LP) in patients with suspected meningitis. A normal CT does not mean that LP is safe. Clinical signs (GCS <12 or fluctuating GCS, papilloedema, bradycardia and hypertension, focal neurology and seizure) are best indicators of when to delay LP. CT findings in meningitis include:

- Often normal.
- May see hydrocephalus.
- Sulcal/cisternal enhancement with contrast.
- Evidence of unequal pressure between intracranial compartments is a contraindication to LP (Fig. 9.8):
  - Lateral shift of midline structures.
  - Effacement of the fourth ventricle.
  - Loss of the suprachiasmatic and basilar cisterns.
  - Effacement of the superior cerebellar and quadrigeminal cisterns with sparing of the ambient cisterns.

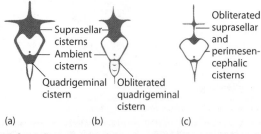

**Fig. 9.8** Suprasellar, perimesencephalic and quadrigeminal cisterns. (a) Normal. (b) and (c) are abnormal.

*MRI*
- Increased signal in the sulci and CSF cisterns on FLAIR.
- Meningeal enhancement on T1W.

## Differential diagnosis

Sulcal high signal on FLAIR is non-specific, other causes include:
- SAH
- Leptomeningeal metastases
- Neurocutaneous melanosis
- Vascular slow flow in acute ischaemic stroke
- Artefact (supplemental oxygen, CSF pulsation, vascular pulsation, motion, susceptibility)

## Complications

- Hydrocephalus.
- Subdural effusion/empyema.
- Cerebral abscess.
- Infarction (secondary to small vessel occlusion).

## Treatment

IV antibiotics (e.g. 2g cefotaxime/ceftriaxone) should be given immediately after LP, or before LP if this will be delayed >30min. Other measures include dexamethasone and management of associated shock/raised ICP.

# Herpes simplex encephalitis

### Aetiology

Herpes simplex type 1 is the commonest cause of viral encephalitis in adults.

### Clinical features

Herpes simplex encephalitis (HSE) presents acutely with headache, fever, mental status change and seizures.

### Imaging

*CT*

- Typically normal for first 3–5 days.
- Low attenuation initially in anteromedial temporal lobe, spreading to insula, subfrontal region and cingulate gyrus. Basal ganglia spared.
- Initially unilateral, becomes bilateral and often asymmetrical.
- Haemorrhage is a late feature.
- Patchy gyral enhancement after IV contrast medium.

*MRI*

MRI is more sensitive and shows abnormalities earlier than CT.
- Restricted diffusion is earliest finding (high signal on DWI, low on ADC).
- Cortical swelling and increased signal on T2W, FLAIR.
- Underlying white matter also involved.
- Foci of haemorrhage appear as low signal on T2*W gradient echo.

### Differential diagnosis

- Limbic encephalitis, a paraneoplastic phenomenon, can appear identical to HSE but is distinguished by its subacute clinical onset
- Low grade glioma
- Acute ischaemic stroke
- Status epilepticus

### Complications

- Memory problems
- Seizures
- Personality change

### Treatment

IV acyclovir should be given if this is suspected clinically, as imaging can be normal at first.

### Further reading

**1.** Joffe AR (2007) Lumbar puncture and brain herniation in acute bacterial meningitis: a review. *J Intensive Care Med* **22**; 194–207.

# ⑦ **Hydrocephalus**

### Definition
Ventricular enlargement caused by an imbalance between CSF production and resorption. It may be 'communicating', with obstruction distal to the outlet foramina of the fourth ventricle, or 'non-communicating', when the obstruction is proximal to these foramina.

### Aetiology
Obstruction to CSF flow from tumour, SAH, meningitis or aqueduct stenosis account for most cases. Rarely due to CSF overproduction by a choroid plexus tumour.

### Clinical features
Headaches, drowsiness, vomiting, neck pain, sixth nerve palsies and papilloedema are amongst the varied presenting features.

### Imaging
#### CT
- Enlarged, 'ballooned' ventricles proximal to level of obstruction.
- All ventricles enlarged in communicating hydrocephalus.
- Periventricular low attenuation in acute hydrocephalus, caused by transependymal leakage of CSF from the ventricle (Fig. 9.9a).
  - Typically more pronounced and confluent than periventricular low attenuation associated with small vessel ischaemia.
- Compression of sulci, effacement of basal cisterns.
- May see enhancing tumour as a cause after IV contrast medium.

#### MR
- Enlarged ventricles as on CT.
- Periventricular halo of high signal on T2W/FLAIR in acute hydrocephalus.
- Corpus callosum thinned and stretched over third ventricle.
- Loss of normal flow void in cerebral aqueduct.

### Differential diagnosis
Ventriculomegaly secondary to loss of cerebral volume, in which the degree of ventricular enlargement is proportionate to the degree of sulcal widening.

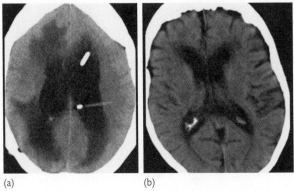

(a)                   (b)

**Fig. 9.9** (a) Periventricular interstitial oedema versus (b) small vessel disease.

### Treatment
Diversion of CSF by external ventricular drainage, ventriculo-peritoneal or ventriculo-atrial shunt. Obstruction at the level of the aqueduct can be treated by endoscopic third ventriculostomy.

# Head and neck

Daniel Scoffings

## :☼: ① **Facial trauma**

### Aetiology
Assault, falls and road traffic collisions are the three most common causes. Alcohol is involved in up to 30% of cases.

### Clinical features
Soft tissue swelling caused by oedema and haematoma can obscure the extent of skeletal deformity. In the acute stage, clinical diagnosis rests on detection of crepitation, abnormal facial mobility and malocclusion.

### Imaging
#### Radiographs
Occipitomental (OM) and 30° angled (OM) views are typically obtained and are the initial imaging modality for uncomplicated facial injuries. For more detailed evaluation, and in the multiply injured patient, CT is recommended.

#### CT
Unenhanced axial CT, which can be obtained as part of a volumetric study incorporating the brain, face and cervical spine in trauma patients (see 📖 p. 54 for indications for C-spine imaging). Images should be reconstructed using a bone algorithm. Axial source images and coronal MPRs are most useful; sagittal MPRs are useful for orbital floor fractures and 3D surface reconstructions are helpful for evaluating complex fractures involving multiple planes.

#### Findings
The facial skeleton can be regarded as a series of buttresses, or regions of increased bone thickness, that provide structural support.

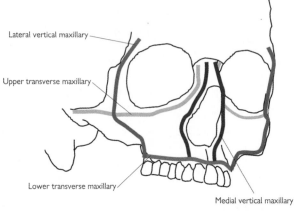

Lateral vertical maxillary

Upper transverse maxillary

Lower transverse maxillary

Medial vertical maxillary

**Fig 10.1** Facial buttresses.

- Upper transverse maxillary:
  - Across zygomatic arch, inferior orbital margin and floor to nasofrontal junction.
- Lower transverse maxillary:
  - Across maxilla above alveolar ridge, posterior extension onto hard palate.
- Medial vertical maxillary:
  - From anterior nasal spine, along margin of nasal fossa, into frontal process of maxilla and nasofrontal junction.
- Lateral vertical maxillary:
  - From posterior maxillary molars, across zygomaticomaxillary suture and body of zygoma and across zygomaticofrontal suture.
- Posterior maxillary:
  - Posterior wall of maxillary antrum, pterygoid process.

### Soft tissue injury
- Subcutaneous oedema/haematoma.
- Sinus haemorrhage.

### Nasal fracture
- Isolated nasal fracture is commonest facial injury (50%).
- 66% due to lateral impact, 16% frontal.
- Most involve the thinner distal third of the nasal bone(s).

### Naso-orbitoethmoid (NOE) fracture (Fig 10.2)
- Disrupts upper part of medial vertical maxillary buttress.
- Fractures of nasal bone, lacrimal bone, frontal process of maxilla, ethmoid air cells, cribriform plate and nasal septum.
- Detaches medial canthal tendon of eyelid, widening distance between inner corners of eyes (telecanthus).
- May disrupt drainage of frontal sinus, leading to mucocele formation.

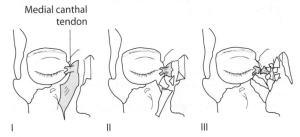

**Fig. 10.2** Classification of naso-orbitoethmoid fractures.

### Orbital fractures
*Medial wall fracture*
- Commonly isolated, also occur with other orbital or facial fractures.
- Orbital emphysema from ethmoid air cells.
- Herniation of fat/medial rectus into defect.
- Differential: congenital dehiscence of lamina papyracea.

*Blow-out fracture*
- Blunt trauma from object too large to enter orbit.
- Orbital floor shattered, usually in middle third; inferior orbital rim usually intact.
- Lamina papyracea also involved in >50%.
- May see herniation of fat/inferior rectus/inferior oblique into maxillary antrum but diplopia can occur without muscle entrapment.
- If inferior rectus retains normal flattened shape, entrapment is unlikely; a rounded shape implies disruption of the fascial sling and possible entrapment (Fig 10.3).

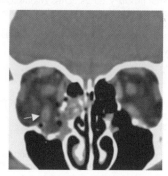

**Fig. 10.3** Blow-out fracture of right orbit with rounded inferior rectus indicating possible entrapment.

⚠ *Trapdoor fracture*
- Inferior rectus trapped beneath orbital floor fragment, which 'hinges' back into normal position.
- Usually in children.
- Needs urgent treatment to prevent motility problems.

**Zygomaticomaxillary complex (ZMC) fractures (Fig. 10.4)**
- Disrupts upper transverse and lateral vertical maxillary buttresses.
- Fractures across zygomaticomaxillary, zygomaticofrontal and zygomaticotemporal sutures, and posterolateral wall of maxillary antrum.
- Often referred to as a 'tripod fracture', although there are typically four fracture lines.

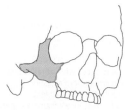

**Fig. 10.4** Zygomaticomaxillary complex fracture.

## Le Fort fractures

- Fracture of pterygoid plate or pterygomaxillary junction is a key finding and best seen on coronal images.
- Each Le Fort injury has a unique component that allows its differentiation from the others (Fig. 10.5):
  - Le Fort I: anterolateral margin of nasal fossa.
  - Le Fort II: inferior orbital rim.
  - Le Fort III: zygomatic arch.

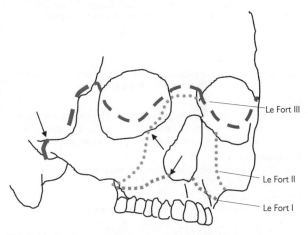

**Fig. 10.5** Le Fort fractures and their unique components (arrows).

- Absence of unique component excludes that particular Le Fort fracture.
- Le Fort injuries of different types can coexist in the same patient, and may co-exist with other facial fractures.
- They can be unilateral.
- Le Fort II and III fractures are associated with intranasal haematoma that can cause asphyxia.

### Treatment

Restoration of occlusion and facial form is the aim. This can require internal fixation with plates and screws. Definitive treatment is often delayed for several days to allow soft tissue injuries to subside. If treatment is delayed beyond one week, the risk of fibrous fixation is increased.

### Further reading

**2.** Hopper RA, Salemy S and Sze RW (2006) Diagnosis of midface fractures with CT: what the surgeon needs to know. *RadioGraphics* **26**; 783–93.

**2.** Rhea JT and Novelline RA (2005) How to simplify the CT diagnosis of Le Fort fractures. *AJR* **184**; 1700–5.

# ① Orbital cellulitis and abscess

### Aetiology
Most cases are secondary to acute sinusitis, the ethmoid air cells are the commonest source.

### Clinical features
Patients present with fever, orbital erythema and oedema, proptosis and pain. Visual disturbance is present in up to 30%. Progression can be rapid, with risk of blindness. **Imaging is therefore a matter of urgency.**

### Imaging
#### CT
*Protocol*

Unenhanced and contrast-enhanced axial CT with coronal reformats. Reconstruct images with soft tissue and bone algorithms.

*Findings*

The periosteal lining of the bony orbit reflects anteriorly onto the tarsal plates as the orbital septum. This divides the orbit into an anterior pre-septal compartment and a posterior post-septal compartment.

#### Pre-septal cellulitis
- Swelling of preseptal soft tissues (eyelids), may extend onto face.
- Post-septal compartment not involved.

#### Post-septal cellulitis
- Pre-septal inflammatory changes usually also present.
- Post-septal, extra-conal inflammation:
  - Stranding of extra-conal fat.
  - Medial extra-conal soft tissue mass (phlegmon).
- Thickening of medial rectus.
- Proptosis.
- Intra-orbital gas may be present.
- Opacification of ethmoid air cells.
  - May see dehiscence of lamina papyracea.

#### Subperiosteal abscess
- Medial extra-conal low attenuation fluid collection with enhancing rim.
- Displaces medial rectus.

### Complications
- Superior ophthalmic vein thrombosis.
- Cavernous sinus thrombosis:
  - Expansion of cavernous sinus
  - Irregular filling defects (NB foci of fat attenuation in the cavernous sinus are normal).
- Intracranial extension:
  - Subdural empyema (low attenuation collection with enhancing rim)
  - Cerebritis or brain abscess.

## Management

Intravenous antibiotics may be successful in less severe cases of orbital infection. Abscesses require surgical drainage.

# ! ? Deep neck space infection

## Aetiology

The commonest causes are tonsillitis and dental infection. Risk factors include diabetes mellitus and IV drug misuse. *Staphylococcus aureus*, streptococci and anaerobes are the most frequent causative organisms.

## Clinical features

Patients typically present with fever, sore throat, odynophagia, neck swelling and lymphadenopathy.

## Imaging

### CT

CECT has high sensitivity but low specificity. Imaging should be obtained from skull base to carina because of the risk of mediastinitis.

### Findings

### General

- Commonest sites are:
  - Parapharyngeal space (67%)
  - Submandibular space (49%)
  - Retropharyngeal space (20%)

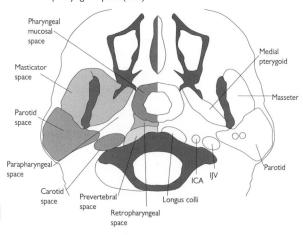

**Fig. 10.6** Deep neck spaces at the level of the oropharynx.

- Abscess suggested by:
  - Rim enhancement around low attenuation centre
  - Irregular, scalloped margin (relatively late finding)
  - Air–fluid level
  - Subcutaneous air

- Attenuation values alone do not reliably distinguish abscess from phlegmon
- Low attenuation areas less than 2ml in volume are unlikely to yield pus
- Lymphadenopathy

*Tonsillar abscess*
- Enlarged tonsils with low attenuation centre and rim enhancement
- Indistinct surrounding tissue planes
- May extend to parapharyngeal, submandibular or masticator spaces

*Retropharyngeal abscess*
- Distension of retropharyngeal space by fluid attenuation material
- Flattening of prevertebral muscles.
- May be mimicked by retropharyngeal oedema, as seen in:
  - Longus colli calcific tendonitis
  - Internal jugular vein (IJV) thrombosis
  - Pharyngitis

*Masticator space abscess*
- Look for destruction of mandibular cortex and periosteal reaction.

## Complications
- Airway compromise
- Mediastinitis
- IJV thrombosis
- Carotid pseudoaneurysm

## Management
- Secure airway with tracheostomy if there is compromise
- Empirical therapy with broad-spectrum IV antibiotics
- Surgical incision and drainage is cornerstone of abscess management
- Percutaneous, imaging-guided catheter drainage may be appropriate in selected cases of unilocular abscesses in patients without airway compromise

## Further reading
**1.** Smith, JL III, Hsu JM and Chang J (2006) Predicting deep neck space ascesses using computed tomography. *Am J Otolaryngol* **27**; 244–47.

# ⑦ Salivary gland infection

### Aetiology

Most infections are viral and produce non-specific imaging findings of glandular enlargement and slight increases in attenuation on CT and heterogeneous areas of low reflectivity on US. Bacterial infections are most often due to *Staph. aureus*, streptococci and *H. influenzae*. Predisposing factors include calculi, dehydration, abdominal surgery, radiotherapy and drugs that reduce salivary flow.

### Clinical features

Ascending infections are more common in the parotid than the submandibular or sublingual glands. Patients present with a swollen, painful, erythematous gland.

### Imaging

#### US

*Protocol*
- 7.5–12MHz linear array transducer.
- Assess gland in two planes, examine whole neck for lymphadenopathy.

*Findings*
- Enlarged gland of reduced reflectivity.
- Multiple small oval areas of low reflectivity may be present.
- Increased vascularity on colour/power Doppler.
- Enlarged lymph nodes (intraparotid/cervical).
- Abscess:
  - Low or absent reflectivity with distal acoustic enhancement.
  - Ill-defined margins.
  - Internal debris, which may be mobile.
  - Hyperreflective foci of gas microbubbles may be present.
- Calculi in Stensen's (parotid)/Wharton's (submandibular) ducts and/or central ducts:
  - Highly reflective foci with distal acoustic shadow.
  - Proximal duct dilatation.

#### CT

More sensitive than US for clusters of salivary calculi. If calculi are suspected, initial scan should be unenhanced as enhancing vessels can mimic small calculi. Give contrast if abscess or other inflammatory process is suspected (100ml of 300mg I/ml at 2–3ml/s, image at 40–50s delay). Angle gantry parallel to the teeth to reduce artefact from dental amalgam.

*Findings*
- Dilated central ducts in early infection
- Enhancement of duct walls
- Calculi in Stensen's/Wharton's ducts and/or central ducts
  - 80–90% calculi occur in submandibular gland
  - Multiple in 25%

- Enlargement of gland.
- Increased attenuation of gland on unenhanced CT.
  - Parotid attenuation normally less than or equal to muscle.
  - Submandibular gland normally isointense to muscle.
- Diffuse glandular enhancement after contrast.
- Enlarged intraparotid or periparotid lymph nodes.
- Abscess formation:
  - Low attenuation centre, enhancing rim.
  - Inflammatory stranding in periglandular fat.
  - Thickening of overlying skin if cellulitis present.

**Further reading**

1. Yousem, DM, Kraut MA and Chalina AA (2000) Major salivary gland imaging. *Radiology* **216**; 19–29.

2. Bialke EJ, Jakubowski W, Zajkowski P et al. US of the major salivary glands: anatomy and spatial relationships, pathologic conditions, and pitfalls. *RadioGraphics* **26**; 745–63.

# Musculoskeletal

# General principles of fracture imaging

## Imaging

### Radiographs

These are sensitive and readily available. It is the initial imaging modality used in the assessment of trauma. At least two views should be obtained in most cases of suspected bone injury.

### CT

CT can better define injuries with complex fracture patterns, and identify intra-articular fracture fragments which can be important for surgical management. Modern multislice CT scanners can provide fast acquisition of isotropic volumetric data, minimizing motion artefacts and allowing reconstruction in the coronal and sagittal planes without loss of resolution. It is more difficult to detect solely trabecular, undisplaced fractures (e.g. some scaphoid fractures) with CT compared to MRI.

Where possible, the patient should be positioned so that the extremities can be scanned in a plane that does not include the rest of the body to minimize beam-hardening artefacts (e.g. holding the arm outstretched over the head). Images should be obtained with bone (e.g. window 2500/500HU) and soft tissue (e.g. window 300/50HU) reconstruction kernels. Thin sections as low as 0.5mm are routine in many centres. 3D volume rendering is a useful feature for some clinicians to help with pre-operative planning. CT images should be reviewed on both bone and soft tissue windows as diverse pathology can be present, e.g. pneumothorax, sternal fracture, bladder rupture. The scout image should also be scrutinized as it provides an additional global view.

### MRI

MRI is not required for most fractures. It is mainly used to evaluate soft-tissue injuries, such as to the surrounding ligament or tendon, or to exclude occult fractures. MRI is very sensitive at detecting bone marrow abnormalities such as bone contusions or solely trabecular fractures.

Given that MRI has a significantly longer imaging time than CT it is often not practical in the emergency trauma setting, particularly when movement artefacts are likely. In addition, any contraindication to MRI may not be known (e.g. ferrous metal foreign bodies).

### Bone scintigraphy

Bone scintigraphy is useful in the assessment of stress fractures. It also has a role in detecting occult fractures, although there is an increasing preference to use cross-sectional imaging modalities (CT, MRI) due to their improved anatomical information and to the relative non-specificity of scintigraphy. Local availability of each modality will usually determine the imaging strategy used.

## Further reading

1. Resnick R and Kransdorf MJ (eds) (2005) *Bone and Joint Imaging*. Elsevier, Philadelphia, PA.

2. Lee JKT, Sagel SS, Stanley RJ and Heiken JP (eds) *Computed Body Tomography with MRI Correlation*. Lippincott William and Wilkins, Philadelphia, PA.

# :✪: ① **Cervical spine trauma**

### Aetiology and epidemiology

Up to 10% of unconscious patients from an RTA or fall have a serious injury to the cervical spine. About 50% of cervical spine injuries occur at C6/7; about 30% occur at C2.

### Clinical features

Localized pain and restricted range of motion. Neurological deficits if there is cord injury.

### Classification

#### C1; atlas

*Jefferson's fracture (unstable; Fig. 11.1)*

This is a burst fracture of C1 from axial loading. There is outward displacement of the lateral masses with fractures of the anterior and posterior arches. Marked prevertebral swelling is often present.

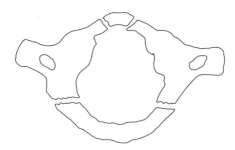

**Fig. 11.1**

*Posterior arch fracture (stable)*

Isolated fractures (unilateral or bilateral) of the posterior arch of C1 occur from hyperextension. Care should be taken to avoid diagnosing a fracture with a congenital cleft of the posterior arch (midline defect with smooth corticated margins).

#### C2; axis

*Odontoid process fractures (types II and III are unstable; Fig. 11.2)*

Type II fractures are the most common and are associated with non-union.

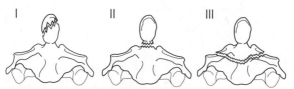

**Fig. 11.2** Classification of odontoid process fractures: type I (avulsion fracture at the tip of the dens; should be differentiated from an os odontoideum), type II (fracture at the base of the dens), and type III (fracture extends into the body of C2).

*Hangman's fracture (unstable) (Fig. 11.3)*
This consists of bilateral fractures of the pars interarticularis of C2 from hyperextension. Anterior subluxation of the C2 body on C3 increases the risk of spinal cord injury.

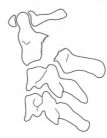

**Fig. 11.3** Hangman's fracture.

*Lower cervical spine fractures*

*Hyperextension injuries*
*Hyperextension dislocation (unstable) (Fig. 11.4)*
There is injury to the anterior longitudinal ligament with disc disruption or an avulsion fracture at the anteroinferior margin of the vertebral body at the attachment of the annulus. This avulsion fragment is typically larger in width than height. Severe neurological deficit is often present. If there is no fracture, this injury can be difficult to detect with radiographs or CT with only prevertebral swelling present.
*Extension teardrop fracture (unstable in extension) (Fig. 11.5).*
This is an avulsion fracture at the anteroinferior margin of the vertebral body. The avulsion fragment is usually small (less than 25% of the AP vertebral body dimension) and typically larger in height than width. Neurological deficit is not usually present.

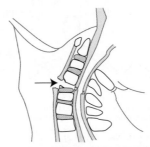

**Fig. 11.4** Hyperextension dislocation. The avulsion fragment is typically larger in width than height.

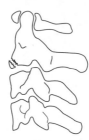

**Fig. 11.5** Extension teardop fracture. The avulsion fragment is typically larger in height than width.

### *Flexion injuries*
*Hyperflexion sprain*
This is a distracting injury to the posterior ligaments, usually without a fracture. Radiographs are frequently normal; occasionally widening of the interspinous distance with localized kyphosis is present. Chronic pain and instability can occur with conservative management.
*Wedge fracture*
See 📖 p. 262.
*Bilateral facet joint dislocation (unstable)* (Fig. 11.6)
This occurs from a high-magnitude flexion injury with ligamentous disruption particularly to the middle and posterior spinal columns. Neurological deficit (narrowing of the spinal canal) and vertebral artery injury is common. Radiographs typically show anterior displacement of the upper vertebra by more than 50% of the AP vertebral body dimension.
*Flexion teardrop fracture (unstable)* (Fig. 11.7)
This occurs from a high-magnitude flexion injury resulting in a large anteroinferior fracture fragment of the vertebral body and posterior ligamentous disruption (widening of the interspinous distance). The fracture fragment is typically 30 to 50% of the vertebral body. Neurological deficit is common.

*Clay-shoveller's fracture (stable)* (Fig. 11.8)
This is an avulsion fracture of the spinous process at the attachment of the supraspinous ligament. It usually occurs at C6 to C7.

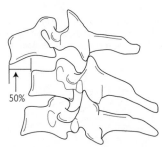

**Fig. 11.6** Bilateral facet joint dislocation. There is usually anterior displacement of the upper vertebra by more than 50% of the AP vertebral body dimension.

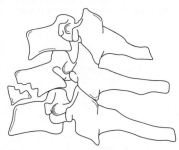

**Fig. 11.7** Flexion teardrop fracture. The fracture fragment is typically 30 to 50% of the vertebral body.

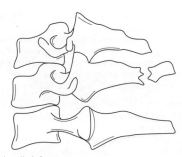

**Fig. 11.8** Clay-shoveller's fracture.

*Compression injuries*
*Burst fracture*
📖 p. 262.

*Flexion–rotation injuries*
*Unilateral facet joint dislocation (stable) (Fig. 11.9)*
Radiographs typically shows anterior displacement of the upper vertebra by less than 50% of the AP vertebral body dimension. Neurological deficit may be present.

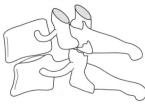

**Fig. 11.9** Unilateral facet joint dislocation. There is usually anterior displacement of the upper vertebra by less than 50% of the AP vertebral body dimension.

## Imaging
In general, radiographs should be obtained in patients with neurology, neck pain or tenderness, or a distracting injury. The Canadian cervical spine rules or the NEXUS criteria (see box below) are decision protocols to exclude significant cervical spine pathology in low-risk patients. There is still debate as to which is more useful in terms of clinical performance. NICE (National Institute for Health and Clinical Excellence, UK) have issued guidelines based on the above two protocols (see box).

### Canadian C-spine rules for clearing low-risk patients with suspected cervical spine injury

Patients must:
• Be alert (GCS 15), not intoxicated or with a distracting injury (e.g. long bone fracture, large laceration).
• Not be at high risk (age 65 or older, dangerous mechanism of injury or paraesthesia in extremities).
• Have a low risk factor (rear-end collision, ambulation at any time post-trauma, delayed onset of neck pain, absence of midline cervical tenderness, can maintain seated position in emergency department) that allows safe assessment of range of motion.
• Be able to actively rotate neck 45° right and left.

### National Emergency X-Radiography Utilization Study (NEXUS) criteria for clearing low-risk patients with suspected C-spine injury

Patients must:
• Be alert (GCS 15), not intoxicated or with a distracting injury.
• Have no midline cervical tenderness.
• Have no focal neurological deficit.

**NICE guidelines 2007**

Patients should have plain radiography of the C-spine with any of the following:

- Neck pain or midline tenderness with: age 65 or older, or dangerous mechanism of injury.
- Unsafe to assess neck movement for reasons other than those above.
- Cannot actively rotate the neck 45° to the left or right.
- An urgent definitive diagnosis of C-spine injury is needed, e.g. pre-surgery
- It is considered safe to assess neck movement if the patient has a low risk factor (see above).

### Radiographs

*Protocol*

AP (full cervical spine), AP (peg) and lateral views are commonly obtained. The lateral view should demonstrate the top of the T1 vertebral body.

The patient should not be placed in a position that would increase the risk of neurological deficit, e.g. log-rolling and a cervical collar should be considered.

*Findings*

- A: check adequacy and alignment (anterior vertebral body line, posterior vertebral body line, spinolaminar line, and spinous process line; clivus baseline) (Fig. 11.10).
- B: check bones, i.e. vertebral body height, fracture.
- C: check cartilage (discs) for uniform disc height.
- S: check soft tissues. Prevertebral swelling is an important indirect indicator of cervical trauma (more than 7mm or 1/3 vertebral body width at C1–4; more than 22mm or 1 vertebral body width at C5–7 is abnormal). The distance between the dens and C1 should be less than 3mm in adults and 5mm in children.
- The three spinal columns (anterior, middle, posterior) should be assessed (Fig. 11.11). Injuries involving more than one column are considered unstable.

### CT

CT is indicated if there is a questionable abnormality on the radiographs or significant clinical concern despite normal plain radiographs. CT is also useful in evaluating the posterior elements or fractures with complex patterns. The entire cervical spine (base of skull to T1) is usually imaged; consider scanning down to T4 in unconscious patients.

### MRI

MRI is used for assessing the cord and adjacent soft tissues. Adding a fat-suppressed sequence (e.g. STIR) helps in detecting these soft tissue injuries (cord, ligaments, intervertebral discs) and assessing if changes to a vertebral body are acute (high signal on fluid-sensitive sequences) or chronic (lack of high signal on fluid-sensitive sequences).

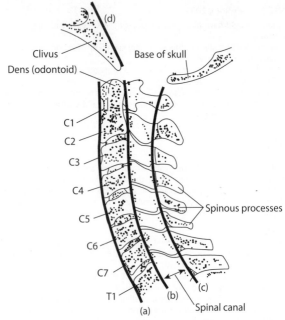

**Fig. 11.10** Lateral view of the cervical spine. (a) Anterior vertebral body line; (b) posterior vertebral body line; (c) spinolaminar line; (d) clivus baseline.

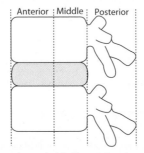

**Fig. 11.11** Denis three-column principle. The anterior column consists of the anterior longitudinal ligament and the anterior half of the vertebral body. The middle column includes the posterior longitudinal ligament and the posterior half of the vertebral body. The posterior column consists of the posterior bone arch and its ligaments.

**Differential diagnosis**
Soft tissue injuries.

**Complications**
- Injuries to the cord and ligaments
- Epidural haematomas
- Vertebral artery dissection

**Further reading**

**1.** Raby N, Berman L and de Lacey G (2005) *Accident and Emergency Radiology: A Survival Guide.* Saunders, USA.

**2.** Resnick R and Kransdorf MJ (eds) (2005) *Bone and Joint Imaging.* Elsevier, Philadelphia, PA.

**3.** Lee JKT, Sagel SS, Stanley RJ and Heiken JP (eds) *Computed Body Tomography with MRI Correlation.* Lippincott William and Wilkins, USA.

**4.** NICE (2007) *Head Injury: Triage, Assessment, Investigation and Early Management of Head Injury in Infants, Children and Adults.* Clinical Guidelines from the National Institute for Clinical Excellence, CG56, available at http://www.nice.org.uk/nicemedia/pdf/cg56NICEGuideline.pdf.

## ✿ ① **Thoracolumbar spine trauma**

### Aetiology and epidemiology

The thoracolumbar junction is a common site for spinal fracture due to its wide range of motion. Most injuries are secondary to flexion or compression forces.

### Clinical features

Localized pain and deformity. Neurological deficits if there is cord injury.

#### Wedge (compression) fracture (Fig. 11.12)

There is typically loss of height of the anterior vertebral body with preservation of the middle and posterior spinal columns. The posterior vertebral wall is intact with no posterior displacement of bone fragments. Severe wedge fractures are associated with injury to the posterior ligaments (demonstrated by widening of the interspinous distance).

#### Burst fracture

This is typically a vertically oriented fracture of the vertebral body with disruption of the posterior vertebral wall and retropulsion of bone fragments into the spinal canal. It is associated with fractures of the posterior elements.

#### Chance fracture seat-belt injury

This is typically a horizontally oriented fracture through the spinous process, pedicles and vertebral body. It occurs from flexion at the thoracolumbar region (level of a seat-belt) which results in distraction of the posterior elements. Significant intra-abdominal injury (e.g. to the small bowel or pancreas) is present in up to 50%.

#### Fracture–dislocation (unstable)

This is intervertebral subluxation or dislocation from disruption of all three spinal columns. Spinal cord injury is often present.

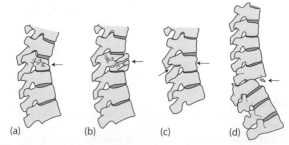

**Fig. 11.12** Simplified diagrams of (a) wedge fracture, (b) burst fracture, (c) chance fracture and (d) fracture-dislocation of the spine.

### Imaging

The three spinal columns (anterior, middle, posterior) should be assessed. Injuries involving more than one column are considered unstable.

#### Radiographs

*Protocol*

AP and lateral views. The patient should not be placed in a position that would increase the risk of neurological deficit, e.g. log-rolling and a spinal board should be considered.

*Findings*

- Assess alignment and vertebral body height. Check the interpediculate distance (AP view) and the posterior vertebral body margin (lateral view). The interpediculate distance should get wider as you go down the spine.
- Adjacent localized haematoma can be detected by deviations of the paraspinal lines (Fig. 11.13).

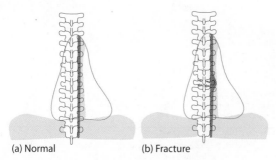

(a) Normal          (b) Fracture

**Fig. 11.13** Localized bulging of the paraspinal lines can indicate a haematoma from an adjacent fracture.

#### CT

CT is useful in evaluating the posterior elements for fractures with complex patterns. Images should contain at least one full vertebra above and below the fracture. Check for any retropulsed bone fragment that may potentially be impinging on the cord.

#### MRI

MRI is used for assessing the cord and adjacent soft tissues ( p. 226; CNS chapters). Adding a fat-suppressed sequence (e.g. STIR) helps in detecting these soft tissue injuries (cord, ligaments, intervertebral discs) and assessing if changes to a vertebral body are acute or chronic.

### Differential diagnosis

- Soft tissue injuries

### Complications

- Injuries to the cord and ligaments
- Epidural haematomas

## Further reading

**1.** Raby N, Berman L and de Lacey G (2005) *Accident and Emergency Radiology: A Survival Guide.* Saunders. USA

**2.** Resnick R and Kransdorf MJ (eds) (2005) *Bone and Joint Imaging.* Elsevier, Philadelphia, PA.

**3.** Lee JKT, Sagel SS, Stanley RJ and Heiken JP (eds) *Computed Body Tomography with MRI Correlation.* Lippincott William and Wilkins. USA

# ① ⑦ Discitis

### Aetiology and epidemiology

Discitis and vertebral osteomyelitis often occur together. The thoracic and lumbar spine are most commonly affected. The routes of infection include haematogenous (e.g. in drug abusers or the immunocompromised) and ascending spread (via the Batson plexus from pelvic infections), and direct implantation.

### Clinical features

Back pain with systemic symptoms of fever and weight loss. Onset is often slow and insidious, and diagnosis can be delayed for many months.

### Imaging

MRI is the preferred imaging modality for suspected spinal infections.

#### Radiographs

*Protocol*

AP and lateral views.

*Findings*

- Abnormalities are usually not visible until several weeks after the onset of symptoms.
- There is typically rapid loss of disc space with destruction of the adjacent endplates.
- Late changes: bone sclerosis and spinal subluxation. TB is slower in progression compared to pyogenic organisms. With TB, there is typically preservation of disc spaces, calcified soft tissue abscesses and lack of severe bone sclerosis.

#### MRI

*Protocol*

- T1; T2 FS (or STIR); T1 FS+Gd.
- Axial and sagittal planes.

*Findings*

- T1: The involved disc and adjacent vertebrae are low in signal. The adjacent endplates are indistinct or destroyed.
- T2: The involved disc and adjacent vertebrae are high in signal (Fig. 11.14).
- T1+Gd: Epidural abscesses have wall enhancement and can be separated from the adjacent thecal sac. There is also enhancement of the disc and adjacent vertebrae.
- Check for extension into the paraspinal soft tissues.

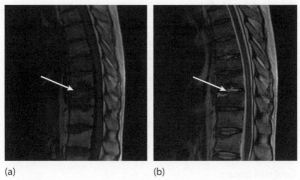

(a)                                    (b)

**Fig. 11.14** (a) Sagittal T1 MR image. Discitis of T10/11 (arrow) with osteomyelitis. The adjacent T10 and T11 vertebrae are hypointense. (b) Sagittal T2 MR image. The infected T10/11 disc (arrow) is hyperintense.

### CT
CT is less sensitive than MRI for spinal infections. It can detect paravertebral soft tissue involvement but is poor for visualizing epidural or subdural spread.

### Nuclear medicine
Radionuclide imaging is used when there are no localizing symptoms. It has a high sensitivity for spinal infections shortly after the onset of symptoms. Bone scintigraphy using MDP labelled with Tc99m is most often used.

**Differential diagnosis**
- Inflammatory spondylitis.
- Spinal tumours.

**Management**
- Intravenous antibiotics.
- Immobilization.

**Complications**
- Neurological deficits occur in up to 40% of patients.

**Further reading**
**1.** Raby N, Berman L and de Lacey G (2005) *Accident and Emergency Radiology: A Survival Guide.* Saunders USA.

**2.** Lee JKT, Sagel SS, Stanley RJ and Heiken JP (eds) *Computed Body Tomography with MRI Correlation.* Lippincott William and Wilkins.

# ☼ ① Skull fractures

### Clinical features

Most present without any neurology. May have loss of consciousness particularly with associated intracranial injury. Basal skull fractures have characteristic signs: CSF leak from the nose or ears, raccoon eyes (bruising around the eyes), and Battle's sign (bruising over the mastoids).

### Classification

#### Undisplaced linear skull fracture

These are the most common type of skull fracture. They can cause epidural haemorrhage or venous sinus thrombosis if they cross an artery or venous sinus. However, these fractures are usually of no clinical significance.

#### Basal skull fracture

These are usually associated with a dural tear and are typically found at three anatomical sites: temporal bone, occipital condyle, and clivus. Adjacent cranial nerves may be injured.

#### Depressed skull fractures

These comminuted fractures are often located at the frontoparietal bone. When the depressed fragment lies deeper than the adjacent inner table of the skull, surgical intervention is usually required.

See 🕮 p. 240 for facial fractures.

Skull fractures are associated with cervical spine injuries in about 15% of cases.

### Imaging

Evidence-based guidelines indicate that skull radiographs should not be requested for mild head injuries. If there is concern about an intracranial haemorrhage, CT should be requested; any skull fracture can be assessed at the same time.

#### Radiographs
*Protocol*
- Lateral and AP frontal views. The AP is often substituted with an AP axial (Towne's) view with trauma to the occipital bone.

*Findings*
- Fractures are lucent lines with irregular branches. Vascular markings are less lucent with sclerotic margins and have smoothly tapering branches. Suture lines occur in characteristic anatomical locations.
- Depressed fractures appear sclerotic.
- Check for a fluid level in the sphenoid sinus on the lateral view. This finding is suggestive of a basal skull fracture.

#### CT
CT is often requested if there is a clinical concern for intracranial haemorrhage. Any skull fracture present can also be assessed on bone window settings.

**Differential diagnosis**
• Intracranial injury.

**Management**
• Usually conservative, particularly when there is no neurology. Surgery is sometimes required with depressed skull fractures.

**Complications**
• Intracranial injury, particularly haemorrhage.

**Further reading**
**1.** Raby N, Berman L and de Lacey G (2005) *Accident and Emergency Radiology: A Survival Guide.* Saunders. USA

# ⊙ Pelvic fractures

### Aetiology and epidemiology
Pelvic fractures account for about 3% of all fractures. They can occur with minor trauma in elderly individuals or with major injury, e.g. RTA.

### Clinical features
- Pelvic tenderness with pelvic springing.
- Pelvic instability on bimanual compression or distraction.

### Classification
The pelvis is a series of bony rings: the main pelvic ring and two smaller rings formed by the pubic rami (Fig. 11.15). It is unusual to break a ring in only one place and a second fracture or dislocation should be actively sought.

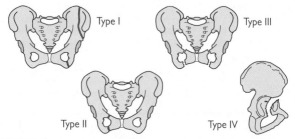

**Fig. 11.15** Kane classification of pelvic fractures: type I (no break to the main pelvic ring), type II (single break), type III (two breaks) and type IV (acetabular fracture).

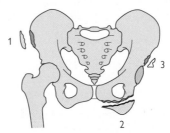

**Fig. 11.16** Tendon insertion sites at various pelvic apophyses. 1 anterior superior iliac spine (sartorius, tensor fascine latae); 2 ischial tuberosity (hamstrings); 3 anterior inferior iliac spine (rectus femoris)

### Type I fractures (stable)
These fractures do not disrupt the main pelvic ring. They include avulsion fractures, single ramus fractures, and isolated fractures of the iliac wing or sacrum; (Fig. 11.16).

### Type II fractures (stable)
These disrupt the main pelvic ring in only one place. They include ipsilateral fractures of both pubic rami and subluxation of the sacroiliac joint or pubic symphysis (may have a fracture nearby). Diastasis of the symphysis pubis greater than 15mm and symphyseal disruption with overlapping of the pubis represent anterior injuries that should strongly raise the possibility of posterior disruption of the pelvic ring.

### Type III fractures (unstable)
These fractures disrupt the main pelvic ring in two places. They include straddle fractures (bilateral fractures involving both pubic rami or dislocation of the symphysis pubis), and Malgaigne's fractures (disruption of both the anterior and posterior pelvic ring). Type III fractures are associated with excessive bleeding, urethral or visceral damage, and nerve damage.

### Type IV fractures (acetabular fractures)
Acetabular fractures occur with impact of the femoral head against the acetabulum especially with posterior hip dislocations (&#x1F4D6; p. 282). Assessment should be made of four bony landmarks: the anterior acetabular rim, the posterior acetabular rim, the iliopubic (anterior) column, and the ilioischial (posterior) column.

## Imaging
### Radiographs
*Protocol*
AP pelvis. Optional views include outlet, inlet and oblique (Judet) views to assess the acetabulum.

*Findings*
- Sacral fractures can be difficult to detect—check that the arcuate lines are not disrupted.
- Avulsion injuries occur in young people and can be recognized from their characteristic location near an apophysis (e.g. ischial tuberosity for the hamstrings, anterior inferior iliac spine for the rectus femoris) (Fig. 11.16).

### CT
CT can evaluate complex fracture patterns such as those involving the acetabulum. CT can also assess injuries to the internal pelvic viscera.

## Differential diagnosis
- Hip fractures
- Injury to the internal pelvic organs

## Complications
Pelvic fractures are associated with major trauma and injuries to the internal pelvic organs are frequent. This includes injury to the:
- Urinary tract
- Pelvic vessels and nerves
- Pelvic viscera

Further radiological assessment is usually done with CT.

## Further reading

**1.** Raby N, Berman L and de Lacey G (2005) *Accident and Emergency Radiology: A Survival Guide.* Saunders, USA.

**2.** Lee JKT, Sagel SS, Stanley RJ and Heiken JP (eds) *Computed Body Tomography with MRI C 2. Bone and Joint Imaging.* Elsevier 2005, USA.

# ! Knee fractures

### Aetiology and epidemiology

Knee fractures are caused by direct or indirect forces.

### Clinical features

Localized pain and swelling at the knee. Inability to straight leg raise with transverse patellar fractures.

### Classification

#### Distal femoral fractures

Usually occur from axial loading with varus or valgus stress. See Fig. 11.17.

#### Patellar fractures

Caused by direct trauma or indirectly from contraction of the quadriceps muscle. Fractures are usually transverse (~50 to 80%) and occur from indirect force.

Care should be taken to avoid diagnosing a fracture with a bipartite patella (a normal variant where there is a separate ossification centre in the superolateral patellar corner).

Dislocations of the patella occur laterally from direct or indirect forces. Predisposing conditions include an abnormally high patella (patella alta) and a shallow femoral trochlear groove. Dislocation is often transient. Axial radiographs may show associated osteochondral fractures of the medial patellar facet and the lateral femoral condyle.

#### Proximal tibial fractures

Tibial plateau fractures (Fig. 11.18) usually occur from valgus stress (e.g. car bumper collision) and often involve the lateral plateau.

#### Proximal fibular fractures

These can occur as part of a Maissoneuve fracture (associated ankle fracture).

Injury to internal soft tissue structures may be present. Fractures of the tibial spine may indicate injury to the cruciate ligaments; an avulsion fracture at the tibial insertion of the lateral collateral ligament (Segond fracture) is strongly associated with an injury to the anterior cruciate ligament.

### Imaging

The Ottawa knee rules provide practical guidelines in selecting patients for radiographs. This consists of any one of:
- Age 55 or over
- Tenderness at the fibular head
- Isolated tenderness of the patella
- Inability to flex to 90°
- Inability to weight-bear both immediately and at assessment for four steps.

### Radiographs

*Protocol*

AP and lateral views are standard. A skyline (axial) view increases detection of patellar fractures. Oblique views can be useful in detecting subtle tibial plateau fractures.

*Findings*

- Some tibial plateau fractures are difficult to detect: look for an area of sclerosis and lateral displacement of the tibial margin.
- A lipohaemarthrosis (Fig. 11.19) indicates an intra-articular fracture.

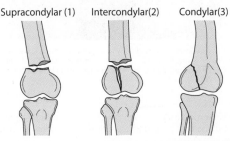

**Fig. 11.17** Distal femoral fractures can be classified as (1) supracondylar, (2) intercondylar, or (3) condylar.

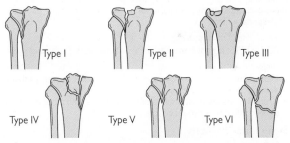

**Fig. 11.18** Schatzker classification of tibial plateau fractures: type I (split fracture of the lateral tibial plateau without depression), type II (split fracture of the lateral tibial plateau with depression), type III (depression fracture of the lateral tibial plateau without splitting), type IV (fracture of the medial tibial plateau; may have split and/or depression), type V (split fracture of the medial and lateral tibial plateaux), and type VI (usually comminuted fracture that separates the articular surface from the diaphysis).

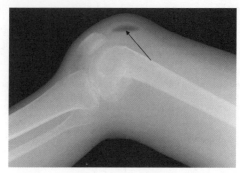

**Fig. 11.19** Lateral knee radiograph showing a lipohaemarthrosis taken with a horizontal beam. A straight fluid line (arrow) is demonstrated at a fat–blood interface (fat above; blood below) indicating the presence of an intra-articular fracture.

## CT
CT can better define injuries with complex fracture patterns, such as fractures of the tibial plateau where articular depression can be difficult to assess with radiographs.

## MRI
MRI is the test of choice for assessing associated injuries to the ligaments, menisci and cartilage. MRI can be used in the acute situation e.g. when there is a suspicion of posterolateral corner injury or if the patient is a professional athlete.

*Protocol (one of many available)*
• PD FS; T2 FS; sagittal plane. T1; T2 FS; coronal plane. T2 FS; axial plane.

*Findings*
• Meniscal tears are linear high signal on fluid sensitive sequences that disrupts an articular surface
• Cruciate tears demonstrate loss of normal fibres with associated high signal on fluid-sensitive sequences.

## Differential diagnosis
• Soft tissue injuries

## Complications
• Neurovascular injury
• Compartment syndrome
• Delayed union/non-union

## Further reading
**1.** Raby N, Berman L and de Lacey G (2005) *Accident and Emergency Radiology: A Survival Guide.* Saunders, USA.

**2.** Resnick R and Kransdorf MJ (eds) (2005) *Bone and Joint Imaging.* Elsevier, Philadelphia, PA.

# ① Shoulder fractures and dislocations

### Aetiology and epidemiology
Proximal humeral fractures usually occur in the elderly. Glenohumeral dislocations are more common in young adults.

### Clinical features
Localized pain and swelling at the shoulder.

### Classification
#### Proximal humeral fractures (Fig. 11.20)
One-part fractures are most common (~80% of proximal humeral fractures).

Fracture-dislocation is a combination of a fracture and the articular surface of the humeral head being displaced outside the joint space.

#### Glenohumeral dislocations
Usually anterior (~90%) and posterior (~4%) dislocations. Inferior, superior and intrathoracic dislocations are rare.

Anterior dislocations are associated with a fracture at the anterior glenoid rim (Bankart) and a fracture at the posterolateral aspect of the humeral head (Hill–Sachs). Posterior dislocations can result from fitting or electrocution injuries and are associated with a fracture at the anterior aspect of the humeral head (reverse Hills–Sachs).

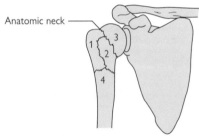

Anatomic neck

**Fig. 11.20** Neer classification system for proximal humeral fractures. The four major segments of the proximal humerus are: 1, greater tuberosity; 2, lesser tuberosity; 3, humeral head; and 4, humeral shaft. Segments are displaced if there is separation by more than 1 cm or angulation by more than 45°. Fractures that do not meet this criteria are considered one-part fractures. There are also two-part (single segment displaced), three-part (two segments displaced) and four-part (all segments displaced) fractures.

#### Acromioclavicular dislocations (Fig. 11.21)
Acromioclavicular joint dislocations account for approximately 10% of all shoulder dislocations.

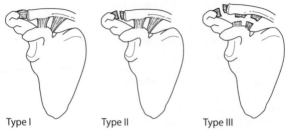

Type I          Type II          Type III

**Fig. 11.21** Simplified classification of acromioclavicular joint injuries: type I (mild sprain of the acromioclavicular ligaments; the coracoclavicular ligaments are intact. Minimal disruption to the acromioclavicular joint alignment); type II (tear of the acromioclavicular ligaments with intact coracoclavicular ligaments; there is a small step or gap at the acromioclavicular joint); type III (tear of both the acromioclavicular and coracoclavicular ligaments; there is frank dislocation at the acromioclavicular joint).

### Traumatic rotator cuff injuries

Rotator cuff injuries occasionally occur from an acute traumatic episode. Plain radiographs are often normal. The diagnosis can be made with ultrasound or MRI, after treatment of the acute symptoms.

## Imaging

### Radiographs

*Protocol*

AP and axillary or scapular Y-views.

*Findings*

- AP view: Check glenohumeral and acromioclavicular alignment, and for glenoid fractures.
- Up to 50% of posterior dislocations are unrecognized on initial presentation. Findings can be subtle on the AP view (lightbulb sign; Fig. 11.22) and are better confirmed on the second view.
- Check for glenohumeral dislocation in the second view.

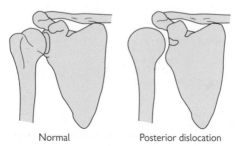

Normal          Posterior dislocation

**Fig. 11.22** Lightbulb sign. The humeral head on the AP view is often internally rotated in posterior glenohumeral dislocation, appearing more rounded like a 'lightbulb'.

## CT

CT can better define intra-articular involvement. It can be useful after reduction of glenohumeral dislocations to assess for associated bone defects (Hills–Sachs, bony Bankart lesions).

## MRI

MRI (with intra-articular contrast medium) is the test of choice for assessing associated glenoid labrum injuries.

*Protocol (*one of many available)
- Dilute gadolinium is injected into the glenohumeral joint
- T1 FS; axial, coronal and sagittal planes. T2 FS (or STIR); coronal plane. T1; axial plane.

*Findings*
- Labral or tendon tears are usually linear high signal on T1 (post Gd) or T2 images.
- Bony deformities are usually best seen on the axial images.

## Differential diagnosis
- Soft tissue injuries

## Complications
- Delayed union/non-union (after fracture)
- Recurrent dislocations (after dislocation)
- Avascular necrosis
- Neurovascular injury (brachial plexus, axillary artery)

## Further reading

**1.** Raby N, Berman L and de Lacey G (2005) *Accident and Emergency Radiology: A Survival Guide.* Saunders, USA.

**2.** Resnick R and Kransdorf MJ (eds) (2005) *Bone and Joint Imaging.* Elsevier, Philadelphia, PA.

# ⓘ **Hip fractures and dislocations**

### Aetiology and epidemiology

Hip fractures can occur with minimal trauma in elderly osteoporotic individuals or with major injury in young adults.

### Clinical features

Localized pain and swelling at the hip.
Inability to move the hip.
Externally rotated and shortened leg.

### Classification

#### *Proximal femoral fractures (Fig. 11.23)*

Intracapsular fractures are approximately twice as common as extracapsular fractures. AVN and non-union are complications associated with intracapsular fractures.

Isolated fractures of the greater or lesser trochanter can occur from avulsion injuries in children or young athletes.

#### *Hip dislocations*

Major trauma is the usual cause of hip dislocations. They can be classified as anterior, posterior (most common) or central, and they can occur with reciprocal acetabular fractures. Posterior dislocations are associated with a flexed knee striking the dashboard during a RTA ('dashboard injury').

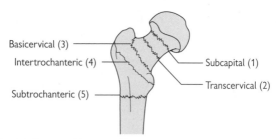

Basicervical (3)
Intertrochanteric (4)
Subtrochanteric (5)
Subcapital (1)
Transcervical (2)

**Fig. 11.23** Fractures of the proximal femur can be classified anatomically as: 1, subcapital; 2, transcervical; 3, basicervical; 4, intertrochanteric; and 5, subtrochanteric. Fractures 1, 2 and 3 are intracapsular, fractures 4 and 5 are extracapsular.

### Imaging

#### *Radiographs*

*Protocol*

AP pelvis and lateral view of the symptomatic hip.

*Findings*

• Some proximal femoral fractures may only be detected as a sclerotic line. Check for associated acetabular and pubic ramus fractures. MRI should be considered if the patient remains symptomatic with normal radiographs.

## CT

CT can better define intra-articular involvement, and is useful after reduction of hip dislocations to assess subtle fracture patterns, particularly involving the acetabulum.

## MRI

MRI is preferred over CT for detecting a radiographically occult proximal femoral fracture.

*Protocol* (one of many available)
- T1; T2 FS (or STIR); large field of view (include both hips); axial and coronal planes.
- Use a small field of view (e.g. one hip) if detailed assessment of a region is required.

*Findings*
- Fractures are low signal on T1 and T2. There is often surrounding marrow oedema (low signal on T1; high signal on T2).

### Differential diagnosis
- Pelvic fractures.

### Complications
- Delayed union/non-union (after fracture)
- Avascular necrosis
- Neurovascular injury (sciatic nerve with posterior dislocations)

### Further reading
**1.** Raby N, Berman L and de Lacey G (2005) *Accident and Emergency Radiology: A Survival Guide.* Saunders, USA.

**2.** Resnick R and Kransdorf MJ (eds) (2005) *Bone and Joint Imaging.* Elsevier, Philadelphia, PA.

# ⓘ Wrist fractures and dislocations

**Aetiology and epidemiology**
Injuries of the upper limb most commonly involve the wrist. Fractures of the distal radius and ulna are approximately 10 times more frequent than carpal fractures.

**Clinical features**
Usually fall onto an outstretched hand. Localized pain and swelling. Tenderness in the anatomical snuffbox if there is a scaphoid fracture.

**Classification**
*Distal radial and ulnar fractures*
Table 11.1 provides a simplified description of the main fracture types. It is important to describe the number of fracture fragments, the amount of displacement or angulation, and the absence or presence of intra-articular involvement.

**Table 11.1** Fractures of the distal radius and ulna

| Fracture | Characteristics |
|---|---|
| Colles' | Dorsal displacement of the distal fragment |
| Smith's | Volar displacement of the distal fragment |
| Barton's | Fracture extending from the dorsal margin of the radius to the radial articular surface |
| Greenstick | Fracture that involves only one cortex; occurs in children |
| Torus | Fracture that produces buckling of both cortices; occurs in children |

*Carpal fractures*
Scaphoid fractures account for about 65% of carpal fractures and may not be demonstrated on initial radiographs. Most scaphoid fractures occur in the waist (~70%) or proximal pole (~20%) and fractures at these locations potentially compromise the blood flow to the proximal portion (most of the blood supply to the scaphoid enters distally). Proximal fractures have a higher rate of avascular necrosis and non-union. Scaphoid fractures are associated with other fracture–dislocations of the wrist.

Isolated fractures of the other carpal bones are less common. Triquetral fractures typically involve the dorsal aspect and are best seen on lateral radiographs (Fig. 11.24). Hamate fractures may involve any portion of the bone, but fractures involving the hamate hook can be difficult to identify on radiographs.

*Dislocation of the distal radio-ulnar joint*
This can occur with a fracture of the radial shaft (Galeazzi fracture–dislocation; this is an example of looking actively for a second fracture when a fracture involves a bone ring, cf. pelvic fractures, 📖 p. 270) or with a Colles' fracture. The ulna usually dislocates dorsally.

*Carpal instability*

Lunate and perilunate dislocations are uncommon injuries.

- *Lunate dislocation*: the lunate dislocates volarly;
- *Perilunate dislocation*: the lunate remains in alignment with the radius while the other carpal bones dislocate dorsally. Perilunate dislocations are often associated with scaphoid fractures.
- *Midcarpal dislocations*: this represents a combination of the previous two injuries with partial volar tilt of the lunate and partial dorsal dislocation of the other carpal bones (Fig. 11.25).

Scapholunate dissociation is relatively common and is suggested when there is widening between the scaphoid and lunate by more than 2mm (Terry Thomas or Madonna sign).

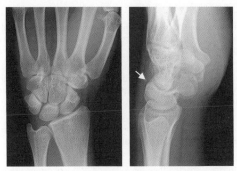

**Fig. 11.24** AP and lateral wrist radiograph. Triquetral chip fracture. There is a small bone fragment (arrow) dorsal to the carpal bones.

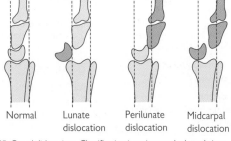

Normal    Lunate dislocation    Perilunate dislocation    Midcarpal dislocation

**Fig. 11.25** Carpal dislocations. Classification is easiest on the lateral view.

## Imaging

### Radiographs

*Protocol*

PA and lateral views. Obtain a scaphoid series (PA, lateral, 45° pronation PA, and ulnar deviation PA) if a scaphoid fracture is suspected.

*Findings*

- PA view: Check for distal radioulnar dislocation, scapholunate widening.
- Lateral view: Check for triquetral fractures, carpal dislocations and that the radial articular surface has its normal palmar tilt.
- If a scaphoid fracture is suspected and the scaphoid series appears normal, *the patient must be re-imaged.* The options include:
  - A repeat scaphoid series in 10–14 days.
  - Bone scintigraphy after 3 days.
  - CT/MRI.
  - MRI is believed to be most sensitive for radiographically occult scaphoid fractures, but the choice often depends on local factors such as cost and availability.

### CT

CT can better define fracture comminution, depression and intra-articular involvement, particularly with the small, complex carpal bones. It can identify occult carpal fractures such as a hook of hamate fracture.

### MRI

MRI is used to evaluate soft-tissue injuries, such as to the triangular fibrocartilage, or to exclude occult carpal fractures.

*Protocol (one of many available)*

If a fracture is suspected then the following protocol can be used: T1; T2 FS (or STIR); coronal plane (additional planes are optional).

*Findings*

- Fractures are low signal on T1 and T2. There is often surrounding marrow oedema (low signal on T1; high signal on T2).

### Bone scintigraphy

Bone scintigraphy can be used to detect radiographically occult fractures such as to the scaphoid. However, there is an increasing preference to use CT or MRI in this situation.

## Differential diagnosis

- Soft tissue injury.

## Complications

- Delayed union/non-union (after fracture)
- Avascular necrosis
- Post-traumatic secondary osteoarthritis
- Neurovascular injury (median and ulnar nerves)

## Further reading

**1.** Raby N, Berman L and de Lacey G (2005) *Accident and Emergency Radiology: A Survival Guide*. Saunders, USA.

**2.** Resnick R and Kransdorf MJ (eds) (2005) *Bone and Joint Imaging*. Elsevier, Philadelphia, PA.

# ① Ankle fractures and dislocations

### Aetiology and epidemiology
Approximately 15% of ankle injuries result in a fracture.

### Clinical features
- Localized pain and swelling at the ankle.
- Inability to weight-bear.

### Classification of fractures
Ankle fractures can be described as unimalleolar, bimalleolar or trimalleolar (involvement of the posterior lip of the tibial plafond). Orthopaedic surgeons make use of the Denis–Weber classification (Fig. 11.26), which is based on the level of the fibular fracture in relation to the syndesmosis.

**Weber A**: Fibular fracture (often transverse) below the syndesmosis. These fractures are usually stable and treated with closed reduction and casting unless accompanied by a displaced fracture of the medial malleolus.
**Weber B**: Fibular fracture (often spiral) at the level of the syndesmosis. Associated injury to the deltoid ligament–medial malleolus complex may be present. These fractures may be stable or unstable depending on the extent of the injury.
**Weber C**: Fibular fracture above the syndesmosis usually associated with injuries to the deltoid ligament–medial malleolus complex and the anterior tibiofibular ligament complex. There may also be injury to the posterior tibiofibular complex.
- *Type C1*: the interosseous membrane is intact and the fracture is low.
- *Type C2*: the interosseous membrane is ruptured at the fracture site
- and the fracture is higher on the fibula.
- *Type C3*: the interosseous membrane is ruptured above the fracture.

The fracture site can be at the proximal fibula (Maisonneuve fracture).
  Weber C fractures are usually unstable and often require open reduction and internal fixation.
  In general, medial malleolar fractures that are displaced and spiral fibular fractures that are above the syndesmosis are considered unstable.

### Other ankle fractures
#### Pilon fracture
This is a comminuted fracture involving the distal tibial articular surface (Fig. 11.27). It results from an axial loading injury. Associated fractures often coexist, e.g. involving the malleoli.

#### Triplane fracture
This usually occurs in adolescents. Fractures are seen in three different axes (planes): a vertical (sagittal) fracture through the distal tibial epiphysis, a horizontal fracture through the distal tibial physis, and an oblique (coronal) fracture posteriorly through the distal tibial metaphysis (Fig. 11.28).

*Juvenile Tillaux fracture*

This usually occurs in adolescents. It is a vertical fracture of the distal tibial epiphysis with lateral extension of the fracture through the open physis and represents a Salter–Harris type 3 fracture (Fig. 11.29).

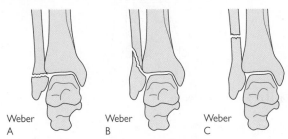

Weber
A

Weber
B

Weber
C

**Fig. 11.26** Denis–Weber classification.

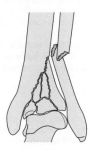

**Fig. 11.27** Pilon fracture.

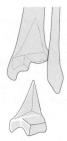

**Fig. 11.28** Triplane fracture (two-part).

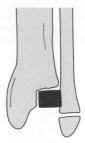

**Fig. 11.29** Juvenile Tillaux fracture.

## Imaging

The *Ottawa ankle rules* provide practical guidelines in selecting patients for ankle radiographs. This consists of pain in the malleolar area with any one of:
- Bone tenderness along the distal 6cm of the posterior edge of the tibia or fibula.
- Bone tenderness at the tip of the medial or lateral malleolus.
- Inability to weight-bear both immediately and for four steps.
- There are additional rules for suspected foot injuries.

### Radiographs
*Protocol*
AP and lateral views are commonly obtained. Some centres make use of the AP mortice view as this can provide better evaluation of the space around the talar dome. The AP mortice view is obtained with the foot internally rotated 20° so that the fibula does not overlap the talus. The lateral view should include the entire calcaneum and ideally include the base of the fifth metatarsal.

*Findings*
- Fractures are usually obvious. Pay particular attention to the talar dome for osteochondral injuries.

### CT
CT can better define injuries with complex fracture patterns, such as triplane or pilon fractures.

### MRI
MRI can be used to assess occult fractures of the talar dome.

### Differential diagnosis
- Ankle ligament sprains.

### Complications
- Delayed union/non-union.

## Ankle dislocations

Ankle dislocations of the tibiotalar joint are usually part of complex malleolar fractures and rarely occur in isolation. Standard radiographs are used to help make the diagnosis. Posterior dislocation of the talus is most common.

Urgent reduction is required.

## Further reading

**1.** Raby N, Berman L and de Lacey G (2005) *Accident and Emergency Radiology: A Survival Guide.* Saunders, USA.

**2.** Resnick R and Kransdorf MJ (eds) (2005) *Bone and Joint Imaging.* Elsevier, Philadelphia, PA.

# ① ② Sternal and rib fractures

## Aetiology
These fractures usually occur from direct blunt trauma, e.g. impact between the sternum and car steering wheel in an RTA. Sternal fractures occur in approximately 5% of blunt chest trauma; rib fractures in 50%.

## Clinical features
Localized pain after direct trauma. Fractures of the first and second ribs imply high-velocity trauma and are associated with injuries to the brachial plexus and subclavian vessels.

## Imaging
### Radiographs
*Protocol*
Sternal views (frontal and lateral).
Routine CXR (frontal and lateral) are usually sufficient for assessing rib fractures. Specific rib views rarely change management.

*Findings*
- The lateral view is most useful for detecting sternal fractures and demonstrating the degree of displacement.
- Most sternal fractures are transverse and occur in the body.
- Look for a flail chest (at least three ribs broken in two or more places).

### CT
*Protocol*
- Chest CT may have been performed to assess for concomitant internal injury but is not indicated to detect rib fractures alone. Use multiplanar reconstructed images with bone settings to assess for skeletal trauma.

*Findings*
- Fractures are more accurately delineated than on plain film.
- Look for associated soft tissue or lung injuries.
- Anterior mediastinal haemorrhage is common with a sternal fracture.
- Assess for upper abdominal organ injuries with lower rib fractures.

## Differential diagnosis and complications
- Cardiac contusion.
- Lung contusion, pneumothorax and flail chest.
- Nerve injuries (e.g. brachial plexus).

## Management
- Conservative management in most cases.
- Early intubation may be required with a flail chest.
- Treat any associated injuries. Assess for cardiac trauma (e.g. elevated troponin levels) with significant displacement of a sternal fracture.

## Further reading
**1.** Miller LA (2006) Chest wall, lung and pleural space trauma. *Radiol Clin North Am* 44; 213–24.

**2.** Bull S (2005) *Skeletal Radiography: A concise introduction to projection radiography.* Toolkit Publications, UK.

# ⚠ Septic arthritis

### Definition and aetiology
Infection in a joint, usually bacterial.

### Clinical features
The joint is usually hot and swollen and typically there is a monoarticular presentation. Pyogenic bacterial infection usually has an acute onset. Involvement with tuberculosis or fungal organisms is more indolent.

Blood tests (CRP, ESR) can be useful. However, joint fluid analysis is more definitive and should be obtained if there is a clinical suspicion of septic arthritis.

### Imaging
Plain radiographs are the initial investigation. If there are typical radiographic findings, joint aspiration and culture should follow. If radiographs are normal, then consider MRI. US is useful to confirm a joint effusion and guide aspiration.

#### Radiographs
*Protocol*
Standard views for the joint in question which usually involve two orthogonal planes.

*Findings*
- Often normal, although peri-articular soft tissue swelling and joint space widening may be seen.
- (*Late changes*) Joint space narrowing and peri-articular erosions which progress to bone destruction. Articular changes occur more slowly in tuberculosis and fungal infection.

#### US
*Protocol*
- A high-frequency (7.5MHz or higher) linear-array transducer can be used to assess most joints, although a lower-frequency probe may be more suitable in obese patients.

*Findings*
- Septic effusions may be completely anechoic or septated/debris-filled.
- Imaging cannot distinguish between inflammatory and infected joint effusions.
- Ultrasound is useful to guide needle aspiration, particularly in paediatric hips.

#### MRI
*Protocol*
- T1; T1 FS+Gd; T2 FS (or STIR).
- Use at least 2 image planes (axial and coronal or sagittal).

*Findings*
- Look for joint effusions, synovial enhancement, marrow changes, cartilage erosion and soft tissue abscesses.

- Reactive bone marrow oedema is present in up to 50% of septic arthritis (in the absence of osteomyelitis).
- MRI is sensitive but not as specific as joint aspiration and the latter is still required to establish the diagnosis.

### Differential diagnosis
- Non-septic arthritis.
- Internal derangement from trauma.

### Management
- Early diagnosis is essential to prevent permanent joint damage.
- Intravenous antibiotics.
- Drainage of joint effusions.

### Complications
- Osteomyelitis
- Joint subluxation and dislocation
- Fibrous or bony ankylosis
- Secondary osteoarthritis

### Paediatric hip pain
Acute hip pain is a common cause of presentation by children to the emergency department. The vast majority of these cases are due to transient synovitis, a self-limiting condition. However, clinical differentiation from more serious conditions such as Perthe's, slipped capital femoral epiphysis or septic arthritis can be difficult. Initial assessment often involves a plain radiograph but findings can be subtle with septic arthritis.

Many centres make use of hip ultrasound to assess for joint effusions. If a joint effusion is present, aspiration is performed under ultrasound guidance and fluid analysis is used to exclude septic arthritis.

### Further reading
**1.** Aurea V, Mohana-Borges R, Chung CB *et al.* (2004) Monoarticular arthritis. *Radiol Clin North Am* **42**; 135–49.

**2.** Berquist T (ed.) (2006) *MRI of the Musculoskeletal System*. Lippincott Williams and WIlkins, Philadelphia, PA.

# ① ⑦ Achilles tendon rupture

## Definition
Complete tear of the Achilles tendon; retraction may be present

## Aetiology and epidemiology
The Achilles tendon is the most commonly injured ankle tendon. Rupture typically occurs in the fourth to fifth decades and with athletic activity ('weekend warriors'). M:F = 5:1. The usual location is 2–6cm above the calcaneal insertion, a region of relative avascularity. Tears at the musculo-tendinous junction are less common but occur with younger people.

## Clinical features
Sudden pain at the back of the ankle during activity. Unable to stand on tiptoes. A tendon gap may be palpable.

Up to 25% of Achilles tendon ruptures can be missed clinically at initial presentation.

The main clinical question is to differentiate complete tears from partial thickness tears or tendinosis (degenerative tendinopathy).

## Imaging
Imaging is helpful when the clinical examination is equivocal or there is a delay in presentation. In particular, imaging is used to differentiate between full- and partial-thickness tears. Ultrasound is the first-line test.

### Radiographs
*Protocol*
Standard AP and lateral views for trauma.

*Findings*
- Loss of the pre-Achilles fat pad.
- Useful to exclude avulsion injuries or other fractures.

### US
*Protocol*
Lie patient in the prone position with the feet hanging over the end of the examination couch. Use a high-frequency (7.5MHz or higher) linear-array transducer with liberal application of US gel over the Achilles tendon. Scan in both longitudinal and transverse planes.

*Findings*
- Full-thickness interruption of the tendon. The space may be filled with fluid or haemorrhage. Look for posterior acoustic shadowing which indicate ruptured tendon ends.
- Measurement of the tendon gap with the foot in plantar flexion is useful to help decide between surgical or conservative treatment.
- Partial-thickness tears and tendinosis demonstrate increased AP tendon diameter. Look for focal defects. At least some intact tendon fibres should be present in partial thickness tears (Fig. 11.30).
- Dynamic tendon movement helps to differentiate full-thickness from severe partial-thickness tears.

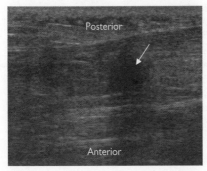

**Fig. 11.30** Longitudinal US image. Partial-thickness tear of the Achilles tendon. There is fusiform tendon swelling with a focal defect (arrow) anteriorly; intact posterior tendon fibres are present.

### MRI
*Protocol*
- Sagittal and axial STIR or PD FS; T1 (any plane).

*Findings*
- Separated tendon ends indicate complete rupture. There is high signal intensity on the fluid sensitive sequences in the tendon gap with acute injuries (Fig. 11.31).
- Partial-thickness tears and tendinosis demonstrate tendon thickening with heterogeneous signal intensity.

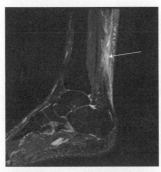

**Fig. 11.31** Sagittal STIR MR image. Rupture of the Achilles tendon. There is complete disruption and retraction of the torn edges of the Achilles tendon with a fluid-filled gap (arrowed).

**Differential diagnosis**
- Partial-thickness tear of the Achilles tendon.
- Tear of the plantaris tendon.

**Management**
- Conservative (leg placed in an equinus cast) or surgical management is based upon the extent of the tear and amount of tendon retraction.

**Complications**
- Achilles tendon re-rupture.

**Further reading**

1. Hartergink P, Fessell DP, Jacobson JA et al. (2001) Full- versus partial-thickness Achilles tendon tears: sonographic accuracy and characterization in 26 cases with surgical correlation. *Radiology* **220**; 406–12.

2. Rosenberg ZS, Breltran J and Bencardino JT (2000) From the RSNA refresher courses. Radiological Society of North America. MR imaging of the ankle and foot. *Radiographics* **20**(Spec no); S153–79.

3. McNally EG (2004) *Practical Musculoskeletal Ultrasound*. Churchill Livingstone, Edinburgh.

# ① ⑦ Intramuscular haematomas

### Definition
Muscle contusion secondary to blunt direct trauma.

### Aetiology and epidemiology
Acute muscle injury is common and accounts for over one-third of all acute sports-related injuries. Direct trauma usually occurs in contact sports and muscles of the lower limb are most often involved.

### Clinical features
Direct trauma to the muscle group with subsequent pain and swelling. There is still residual function unlike a muscle rupture.

### Imaging
The diagnosis is usually made clinically and imaging tends to be reserved for when the diagnosis is in doubt, when the symptoms are not responding to therapy, or if the patient is a professional athlete. US is the first-line investigation. MRI is an alternative.

The appearance of haemorrhage varies with both US and MRI according to its age. Haematoma may predominate within the muscle or lie outside the epimysial covering between muscles. Intramuscular fluid–fluid levels (a layering effect with cellular components of the blood settling depend-ently and the less dense plasma forming a layer on top) may be seen.

#### *Radiographs*
*Protocol*
Standard views as for trauma.

*Findings*
• Useful to exclude a fracture.
• Myositis ossificans may be present, usually 6 weeks after the injury.

#### *US*
*Protocol*
A high-frequency (7.5MHz or higher) linear-array transducer can be used to assess most muscles, although a lower-frequency probe may be more suitable in obese or very muscular patients.

*Findings*
• Acute haematomas (0–4hrs) are echogenic with ill-defined margins and extensive surrounding echogenic swelling of the muscle. Dynamic imaging can help exclude a complete tear.
• After a few days, the haematoma becomes predominantly hypoechoic with a better defined echogenic margin (Fig. 11.32). Over the next few weeks, the echogenic periphery gradually fills in towards the centre. The majority of muscle haematomas from sporting injuries heal with normal muscle regeneration.

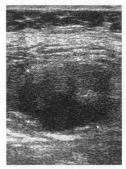

**Fig. 11.32** Longitudinal US image. Rectus sheath haematoma (arrows) which is predominantly hypoechoic with echogenic areas.

### MRI

*Protocol*

Fluid sensitive sequences (T2 FS, STIR) demonstrate oedema well. T1-weighted sequences provide information about subacute haemorrhage and muscle atrophy/fatty infiltration. Use at least two image planes (axial and coronal or sagittal).

*Findings*

- *Acute haematomas* (0–48hrs) are often isointense to skeletal muscle on T1-weighted images and hypointense on fluid sensitive sequences. Adjacent oedema (low signal on T1; high signal on T2) can be a prominent feature.
- *Subacute haematomas* (weeks to months old) usually demonstrate increased signal intensity on both T1- and T2-weighted images due to the presence of extracellular methaemoglobin. As the lesion ages, the wall of the haematoma may become hypointense from haemosiderin deposition and fibrosis.

*Differentiation between a simple haematoma and a haemorrhagic neoplasm can be difficult with imaging.* Administration of contrast medium can help to exclude a neoplasm when the lesion in question shows no enhancement, but usually, correlation with the clinical history is most useful in this context.

Rectus sheath haematomas deserve a special mention. They are uncommon but are often an unsuspected cause of abdominal pain. Ultrasound is again the first-line test. The Valsalva manoeuvre and visualization of a defect in the deep fascia help differentiate from an abdominal wall hernia. Forced expiration against a closed airway increases intra-abdominal pressure and improves detection of abnormal movement of intra-abdominal contents through a deep fascial defect.

### Further reading

1. McNally EG (2004) *Practical Musculoskeletal Ultrasound*. Churchill Livingstone, Edinburgh.

2. Boutin RD, Fritz RC and Steinbach LS (2002) Imaging of sports-related muscle injuries. *Radiol Clin N Am* **40**; 333–62.

# ⊕ ⑦ **Retained foreign body**

### Definition and aetiology

A foreign body retained in the soft tissues is a common scenario in the emergency department, usually involving metal, glass or wood.

### Clinical features

Occurs with penetrating injuries. Patient complains of a stinging sensation deep to a puncture wound. Up to 40% of retained foreign bodies in the soft tissues are overlooked at initial examination. Detection and removal is important to avoid infectious or inflammatory complications.

### Imaging

- Plain radiographs are often the first imaging modality used and are good at detecting metal or glass. They can fail to detect non-radio-opaque foreign bodies such as wood or plastic. Radiographs can also be of limited use for precise localization of foreign bodies situated deep in the tissues.
- Ultrasound is used for detecting non-radio-opaque foreign bodies and accurately localizing all types of soft tissue foreign bodies. A mark can be placed on the skin overlying the foreign body to aid removal with ultrasound guidance or by surgical means.

### *Radiographs*

*Protocol*

Use a soft tissue exposure with at least two projections. The soft tissue should be imaged without overlying bone where possible. Place a skin marker at the site of the puncture wound.

*Findings*

- Radio-opacity in the soft tissues.
- Note that all glass is radio-opaque to some degree on radiographs.

### *US*

*Protocol*

Use a high-frequency (7.5MHz or higher) linear-array transducer with liberal application of US gel. Place the probe gently on the skin.

*Findings*

- Foreign bodies are often echogenic with posterior acoustic shadowing (Fig. 11.33). There may be a surrounding hypoechoic rim of granulation tissue, oedema or haemorrhage.
- Look for associated soft-tissue complications, e.g. soft-tissue abscesses, tendon or neurovascular injuries.

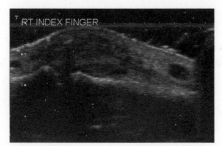

**Fig. 11.33** Ultrasound of a small thorn in the soft tissues of the right index finger. There is an echogenic foreign body (between cursors) with a surrounding hypoechoic region.

## CT or MRI

In exceptionally difficult cases, CT or MRI should be considered. Add a gradient echo sequence to emphasize susceptibility artefacts when looking for metallic foreign bodies with MRI.

## Further reading

**1.** Horton LK, Jacobson JA, Powell A *et al.* Sonography and radiology of soft-tissue foreign bodies. *Am J Roentgenol* 2001; **176**; 1155–9.

**2.** Boyse TD, Fessell DP, Jacobson JA *et al.* US of soft-tissue foreign bodies and associated complications with surgical correlation. *Radiographics* 2001; **21**; 1251–6.

**3.** McNally EG (2004) *Practical Musculoskeletal Ultrasound*. Churchill Livingstone, Edinburgh.

**FURTHER READING**

# Obstetrics, gynaecology, and breast

# ① ⑦ **Haemorrhagic ovarian cyst**

## Aetiology

Due to bleeding into follicular ovarian cyst or corpus luteum cyst.

## Clinical features

Usually affects women of reproductive age. May be asymptomatic or cause acute pelvic pain which usually settles within several hours. Rarely a haemorrhagic cyst can rupture to produce a haemoperitoneum which can be life-threatening, especially in conjunction with anticoagulation. Pregnancy test is negative.

## Imaging

### US

*Protocol*
- Abdominal or pelvic US with curvilinear probe (4MHz adults, 6MHz children). If cystic lesion >3cm, a follow-up ultrasound is recommended in 6 weeks to ensure resolution.

*Findings*
- Ovarian cyst shows lace-like reticular echos or intracystic solid clot.
- Blood flow detected on colour Doppler in 19–61%, does not distinguish haemorrhagic cyst from neoplasm.
- Most helpful features to distinguish from neoplasm are papillary projections and nodular septa in the latter.
- If cyst is ruptured, complex free fluid seen in pelvis/abdomen.
- Over time the appearances of ovarian mass become more cystic with reduction in size of the cyst and complete resolution of cystic mass on average by 4 weeks (2–8 weeks).

### CT

*Protocol*
- Oral contrast medium 90 and 30min prior to the study.
- Unenhanced CT (optional) through abdomen and pelvis followed by portal phase imaging.

*Findings*
- NECT: Mass of heterogeneous attenuation with high attenuation component (45–100HU) in the adnexa. May demonstrate a fluid–fluid level.
  - If cyst rupture, there is a haemoperitoneum seen as fluid of high attenuation.
- CECT: delineates cyst wall (1–10mm) which may show discontinuity.
  - Excludes other causes of haemoperitoneum, e.g. ruptured hepatic adenoma.
  - Delayed CT shows extravasation and collection of contrast medium in pelvis.

### MR

*Protocol*
- T1 axial; T2 axial, sagittal, coronal; T1 axial with fat saturation ± contrast.
- Optional: T2 axial or axial oblique with fat saturation.

*Findings*
- T1: majority of cysts (64%) are hypointense on T1, remainder are intermediate to high signal intensity (SI) in at least a portion of the cyst. Haemoperitoneum appears as fluid hyperintense to urine in the bladder.
- T2: majority are heterogeneous and hyperintense. 18% can be homogenously hyperintense. May get haematocrit effect with hyperintense non dependent layer and dependent hypointense layer.
  - Cyst wall may be thick but smooth and hypointense.
- T1+Gd: wall enhancement.

## Differential diagnosis
- Endometrioma.
- Tubo-ovarian abscess.
- Ovarian cystadenoma/cystadenocarcinoma.
- Ectopic pregnancy.

## Management
- Conservative and supportive therapy with pelvic US follow-up where appropriate.
- Surgery if haemodynamically unstable with massive bleeding.

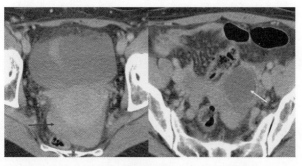

**Fig. 12.1** Axial CECT showing two sections through the pelvis: high attenuation fluid is demonstrated in the Pouch of Douglas (haemoperitoneum, black arrow) due to ruptured haemorrhagic ovarian cyst (white arrow).

## Further reading

**1.** Bennett GL, Slywotzky CM and Giovanniello G (2002) Gynecologic causes of acute pelvic pain: spectrum of CT findings. *Radiographics* **22**; 785–801.

**2.** Nemoto Y, Ishihara K, Sekiya T *et al.* (2003) Ultrasonographic and clinical appearance of hemorrhagic ovarian cyst diagnosed by transvaginal scan. *J Nippon Med Sch* **70**; 243–9.

**3.** Miele V, Andreoli C, Cortese A *et al.* (2002) Hemoperitoneum following ovarian cyst rupture: CT usefulness in the diagnosis. *Radiol Med (Torino)* **104**; 316–21.

**4.** Kanso HN, Hachem K, Aoun NJ *et al.* (2006) Variable MR findings in ovarian functional hemorrhagic cysts. *J Magn Reson Imaging* **24**; 356–61.

# ① ② **Adnexal torsion**

## Definition

Torsion of the ovary, ipsilateral fallopian tube or both around the vascular pedicle, resulting in vascular compromise and haemorrhagic infarction.

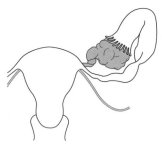

**Fig. 12.2** Torsion of the ovary.

## Aetiology and epidemiology

Usually occurs in the reproductive age group (71% of women between 20–39yrs age). There is a higher incidence in pregnancy. It accounts for 2.7% of all cases with acute abdominal pain in gynaecology. 64–82% of adult cases have a causative finding. Malignancy is found in up to 2% of adult patients. Cystic adnexal tumours are more likely to undergo torsion than solid tumours. Usual causes include benign cystic teratomas, para-ovarian/tubal cysts, follicular cysts, serous or mucinous cystadenomas.

## Clinical features

Sudden onset of abdominal/pelvic pain with nausea and vomiting. Fever and leucocytosis may be present.

## Imaging

### US

*Protocol*
- Abdominal (with full urinary bladder) with curvilinear probe (4MHz) and transvaginal US. Doppler US should also be performed.

*Findings*
- Ovary appears enlarged with multiple peripheral cysts. Cysts may be echogenic if haemorrhage present.
- If underlying lesion, may appear as a septated cystic mass with eccentric wall thickening.
- Tubal thickening if fallopian tube involved.
- Twisted vascular pedicle appears as a round hyperechoic structure with multiple hypoechoic concentric stripes (coiling or target appearance).
- Colour Doppler:
  - flow signal within twisted vascular pedicle identified as 'whirlpool sign'.

- Pulsed Doppler:
  - Early phase: within the torted adnexa, venous flow is decreased and arterial flow shows spiky, high resistance pattern.
  - Later stage, both arterial and venous flows are absent.
  - **NB. The presence of arterial or venous flow does not exclude adnexal torsion!**

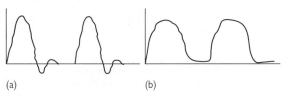

(a)                                          (b)

**Fig. 12.3** Schematic of the pulsed Doppler arterial waveforms in ovarian torsion (a) high resistance; as compared to the normal ovary (b) low resistance.

## CT

*Protocol*
- Oral contrast medium given 90 and 30min before the study.
- Pre (optional) and post iv contrast medium studies (in the portal venous phase) performed through the abdomen and pelvis.

*Findings*
*NECT*
- Tubular solid mass (fallopian tube) noted around adnexal mass.
- Haemorrhage present if attenuation greater than 50 HU.

*CECT*
- Adnexal mass (5–20cm in diameter) is usually cystic ± fat. Otherwise mixed cystic solid or solid lesion. Demonstrates variable enhancement with twisted vascular pedicle.
- Cyst wall thickness average of 10mm with infarction, 3mm without.
- Ascites: >50%.

## MR

*Protocol*
- T1 axial; T1 axial with fat saturation ± contrast; T2 axial, sagittal, coronal.
- Optional: T2 axial or axial oblique with fat saturation.

*Findings*
- Fallopian tube appears as solid mass adjacent to adnexal mass. Haemorrhage is present if high signal intensity on T1 and T2 weighted imaging.
- Adnexal mass has beak-like protrusion at periphery corresponding to twisted pedicle.
  - Torted ovary shows enlarged oedematous stroma which is hyperintense. Follicles are displaced peripherally.

- Cyst wall shows concentric or eccentric thickening.
- Haemorrhage into cyst wall is high signal intensity on T1 and T2 weighted imaging.
- T1+Gd FS: adnexal mass shows variable enhancement with twisted vascular pedicle.

### Differential diagnosis

- Ruptured functional cyst, ectopic pregnancy, pelvic inflammatory disease (PID), haematosalpinx.

### Management

- Laparascopic untwisting in non-infarcted ovary.
- Laparascopic salpingo-oophorectomy in infarcted ovary.
- Any coincidental tumour can be excised at initial presentation or at 2nd laparoscopy.

### Further reading

1. Rha SE, Byun JY, Jung SE et al. (2002) CT and MR imaging features of adnexal torsion. *RadioGraphics* **22**; 283–94.

2. Albayram F and Hamper UM (2001) Ovarian and adnexal torsion: spectrum of sonographic findings with pathologic correlation. *J Ultrasound Med* **20**; 1083–9.

# ⑦ Pelvic inflammatory disease

Laparoscopy is the gold standard for diagnosis. However, imaging is preferred as laparoscopy is an invasive test, requiring general anaesthesia.

## Aetiology and epidemiology

Ascending infection from aerobic and anaerobic organisms, e.g. *Neisseria gonorrhoeae*, *Chlamydia trachomatis*. Risk factors include young age, multiple sexual partners, low socio-economic status, intrauterine contraceptive device and pelvic instrumentation.

## Clinical features

Fever, abdominal/pelvic pain, vaginal discharge, or asymptomatic (≤35%).

## Imaging

MR is more accurate than US in the diagnosis of PID but may be less readily available and is more expensive. CT can determine the extent of involvement and identify complications. Both US and CT can be used for image guided aspiration and drainage.

**Table 12.1**

|  | Sensitivity (%) | Specificity (%) | Accuracy (%) |
|---|---|---|---|
| Transvaginal US[1] | 81 | 78 | 80 |
| Transvaginal US with power doppler[2] | 100 | 80 | 93 |
| MRI[1] | 95 | 89 | 93 |
| CT[3] | 87 | 100 | 98 |

## US

*Protocol*
- Abdominal (4 MHz) with curvilinear probe and transvaginal US.

*Findings*
- Free fluid in pouch of Douglas: this is seen in 50% of patients with PID. Initially small and anechoic. Becomes echogenic and has septations with the presence of pus or blood.
- Endometritis results in increased uterine size. Endometrium becomes echogenic and endometrial cavity is distended with fluid (>14mm). There is an indistinct border between uterus and adnexa.
- Salpingitis: Fallopian tubes become dilated and tortuous and contain fluid which is either anechoic or echogenic due to pus (pyosalpinx) or blood (haematosalpinx). Increased blood flow on Doppler imaging.
  - 'Cogwheel sign': incomplete septa within fallopian tubes.
  - 'String sign' is present in 50% of cases where there is increased interface within Fallopian tube due to exudates.
- Ovaries are enlarged with loss of corticomedullary differentiation.
  - Tubo-ovarian abscess appears as a multi/unilocular complex thick walled cystic mass +/– adhesions.
  - Increased blood flow and low pulsatility index (<1.0) in acute stage.

## CT

*Protocol*

- Portal phase imaging with oral contrast 90 and 30 mins prior to study.

*Findings*

- Early PID: features include pelvic fat stranding, abnormal enhancement of cervix/endometrium with endometrial fluid, enlarged abnormally enhancing ovaries, enhancing thickened fallopian tubes.
- Advanced PID: pyosalpinx appears as enhancing dilated fluid-filled fallopian tube. Tubo-ovarian abscess appears as enhancing uni/multilocular thick-walled cystic mass +/− internal gas bubbles. There may be associated hydronephrosis, serosal thickening of rectosigmoid colon, para-aortic lymphadenopathy, bowel ileus and inflammatory changes in right upper quadrant (Fitz Hugh Curtis syndrome).

## MR

*Protocol*

- T1 axial; T1 axial with fat saturation ± contrast; T2 axial, sagittal, coronal; Optional: T2 axial or axial oblique with fat saturation.

*Findings*

- Fluid in pelvis and endometrial cavity: homogenous/heterogeneous high signal intensity on T2.
- Fallopian tubes are dilated, tortuous and fluid filled (hydrosalpinx). Fluid is heterogeneous high signal intensity on T2. Wall enhancement present in pyosalpinx.
- Tubo-ovarian abscess appears as a cystic solid mass with internal septa and possibly gas, usually of low SI on T1 (with hyperintense inner rim of granulation tissue) and high SI on T2. Wall enhances with gadolinium. Pelvic lymphadenopathy may be present.

## Differential diagnosis

- Ovarian neoplasm, adnexial torsion, haemorrhagic ovarian cyst/endometrioma, pelvic abscess from another cause.

## Management

- Conservative with intravenous antibiotics; removal of intrauterine contraceptive device (IUCD) if present; percutaneous/transrectal drainage of persistent tubo-ovarian abscess; surgical drainage.

## Long-term complications

- Ectopic pregnancy, chronic pelvic pain, infertility.

## Further reading

**1.** Tukeva TA, Aronen HJ, Karjalainen PT *et al.* (19998) MR imaging in pelvic inflammatory disease: comparison with laparoscopy and US. *Radiology* **210**; 209–16.

**2.** Molander P, Sjöberg J, Pavonen J *et al.* (2001) Transvaginal power Doppler findings in laparoscopically proven acute pelvic inflammatory disease. *Obstet Gynecol* **17**; 233–8.

**3.** Rao PM, Feltmate Cm Rhea JT *et al.* (1999) Helical computed tomography in differentiating appendicitis and acute gynecologic conditions. *Obstet Gynecol* **93**; 417–21.

# ! ? Ovarian hyperstimulation syndrome

### Aetiology
Usually iatrogenic secondary to ovarian stimulant drug therapy for infertily; very rarely occurs spontaneously in pregnancy.

### Clinical features
May include abdominal pain, ascites, nausea, vomiting, pleural effusion and hypovolaemia. Occasionally life-threatening.

### Imaging
- Findings similar on US, CT and MRI.
- Bilateral symmetrically enlarged ovaries, containing peripherally placed distended corpora lutea cysts of varying sizes, with 'spoke wheel' appearance. Cyst walls and central stroma enhance on CECT and MRI+Gd.
- +/– ascites, pleural effusions.

### Differential diagnosis
- Endometrioma.
- Bilateral hydrosalpinx.
- Polycystic ovarian syndrome.
- Ovarian cystic neoplasms.

### Management
- Supportive therapy with cessation of infertility drugs.
- Pelvic US follow-up to ensure resolution.

### Further reading
**1.** Bennett GL, Slywotzky CM and Giovanniello G (2002) Gynecologic causes of acute pelvic pain: spectrum of CT findings. *Radiographics* **22**; 785–801.

**2.** Hricak H (ed.) (2007) *Diagnostic Imaging: Gynaecology.* Amirsys-Elsevier.

# ! ? **Problems in early pregnancy**

## Definition

Miscarriage refers to the loss of a pregnancy before 24 weeks. It accounts for around 50 000 inpatient admissions in the UK annually and remains an occasional cause of maternal death.[1] The term 'abortion' is no longer used in the UK to refer to spontaneous pregnancy loss.[2]

## Aetiology

Many early pregnancy losses (miscarriage prior to 12 weeks) occur due to chromosomal abnormalities in the conceptus[3] and are not routinely investigated. Some units recommend investigation for pregnancy loss after 12 weeks' gestation; cases of recurring miscarriage should be investigated according to evidence-based guidelines.[4]

## Clinical features

While most early pregnancy problems are managed in dedicated Early Pregnancy Assessment Units, radiologists will occasionally have to assess women who present with symptoms of bleeding or pain in early pregnancy, and thereby differentiate an ongoing intrauterine pregnancy from a miscarriage or ectopic pregnancy (see 📖 p. 322). Furthermore, the radiologist may be involved in the imaging of women with pain who are unaware that they may be pregnant so the ability to identify an intrauterine pregnancy is of paramount importance.

- Most women will present with vaginal bleeding, abdominal pain or the passage of tissue *per vaginam* (PV).
- The cervix may be open on examination.
- There may be loss of the normal symptoms of pregnancy and fever if complicated by infection.

## Epidemiology

Problems in early pregnancy are very common, affecting 15–20% of clinical pregnancies; many more women will have symptoms suspicious for miscarriage. There is an association with increasing maternal age.

## Non-imaging investigaions

All women of child-bearing age presenting with either pain or bleeding should be assessed for urine and/or serum βHCG (📖 p. 322 for further details). The unstable patient with such symptoms should undergo immediate assessment by an obstetrician/gynaecologist capable of surgical management of miscarriage and ectopic pregnancy.

## Imaging

Transvaginal (TV) US is the mainstay for the investigation of miscarriage. When βHCG is positive and the patient is clinically stable, the role of imaging is to:
- identify any pregnancy,
- identify the site of the pregnancy,
- if intrauterine, determine its viability.

## US

*Protocol*

Although some practitioners may prefer to start with a transabdominal (TA) approach using a curvilinear probe (3–5MHz in adults), TV US is superior in the assessment of early pregnancy complications. Knowledge of the last menstrual period date, and the date of the first positive pregnancy test, may help with the interpretation of the US findings.

A longitudinal (sagittal) section through the uterus should be obtained.

*Findings*

- Demonstrating continuity of the cervical canal, endometrial cavity and the gestation sac confirms that the gestation sac is within the uterine cavity.
- The dimensions and shape of any gestation sac should be recorded.
- The presence of a yolk sac and fetal pole should be recorded with measurements.
- If a fetal heart pulsation is seen, this should also be recorded.
- If the uterus is empty, then a careful search for an ectopic pregnancy should be performed (see 📖 p. 322). If neither an intra- or extra-uterine pregnancy can be identified, this is referred to as 'pregnancy of unknown location' and quantitative serum βHCG would be recommended by many obstetrician/gynaecologists in such circumstances.[5] The finding of a subchorionic haematoma (bleeding between the gestation sac and the endometrium) is common, occurring in around 18% of women presenting with threatened miscarriage. There is no clear association with an adverse pregnancy outcome.
- **In all cases, the findings of the examination should be explained to the woman and appropriate referral or follow-up arranged.**

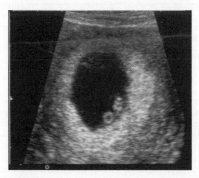

**Fig. 12.4** TAUS: Within the uterus is an ovoid-shaped gestation sac. Within the sac is the ring-like yolk sac, and the adjacent fetal pole. In this case, a fetal heart pulsation could be clearly seen.

## Classification

### Missed miscarriage

If a fetal pole (embryo) is visualized, the crown-rump length is greater than 6mm and no fetal heart pulsation is seen, then a diagnosis of missed miscarriage may be made. Similarly, if no yolk sac or fetal pole is visible and the mean dimensions of the gestation sac are greater than 20mm, a diagnosis of missed miscarriage may be made.

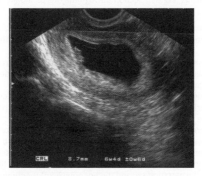

**Fig. 12.5** TVUS of an irregularly shaped gestation sac. There is an indistinct fetal pole measuring 8+mm, but no fetal heart pulsation was seen.

### Pregnancy of uncertain viability

In those pregnancies in which the embryo and sac are smaller than 6mm and 20mm respectively, then a repeat ultrasound scan should be performed at least 1 week later to clarify the diagnosis. This scenario may be referred to as a 'pregnancy of uncertain viability'.

### Complete and incomplete miscarriage

There is a lack of consensus in the criteria used to diagnose either complete or incomplete miscarriage; local guidelines should be used where possible.[5]

Complete miscarriage is usually diagnosed when the endometrium is very thin and regular (typically less than 15mm) and there are no obvious retained products of conception. There is often a history of heavy vaginal bleeding and passage of tissue *per vaginam* which are resolving. Caution must be taken as the appearances of the uterus may be similar in ectopic pregnancy (although usually with a thickened endometrium; 📖 p. 322).[5,6]

Incomplete miscarriage may be diagnosed when there is no evidence of a gestation sac and the endometrial thickness is greater than 15 mm in the antero-posterior plane, with the presence of heterogenous or irregular tissue.[5,6]

## Management

For a non-viable pregnancy, the three main management options are expectant management, medical management (evacuation of the uterus using mifepristone or prostaglandins, e.g. misoprostol) and surgical management (suction evacuation of the uterus).[2,6] In most circumstances, all three options should be available to the woman unless contraindications exist or the unit lacks the facilities to provide one or more of these alternatives.

Women who are Rhesus D negative are normally offered Anti-D prophylaxis if they undergo either medical or surgical evacuation of the uterus, or if they have episodes of vaginal bleeding after 12 weeks' gestation.[2]

## Further reading

**1.** Saving Mothers' Lives (2007), CEMACH London 2007 http://www.cemach.org.uk.

**2.** RCOG (2006) *The Management of Early Pregnancy Loss*. Greentop Guideline 25. Available at http://www.rcog.org.uk/resources/Public/pdf/green_top_25_management_epl.pdf.

**3.** ACOG (1995) Early pregnancy loss. ACOG technical bulletin. *Int J Gynaecol Obstet* **51(3)**; 278–85.

**4.** RCOG (2003) *The Investigation and Treatment of Couples with Recurrent Miscarriage*. Greentop Guideline. Available at http://www.rcog.org.uk/resources/Public/pdf/Recurrent_Miscarriage_No17.pdf

**5.** Condous G (2004) The management of early pregnancy complications. *Best Pract Res Clin Obstet Gynaecol* **18(1)**; 37–57.

**6.** Sagili H and Divers M (2007) Modern management of miscarriage. *The Obstetrician and Gynaecologist* **9**; 102–8.

The guidelines of the Association of Early Pregnancy Units, which include early pregnancy scanning milestones, are available online from http://www.earlypregnancy.org.uk.

## :⚙: ⓘ ⓥ **Ectopic pregnancy**

### Definition and aetiology

An ectopic pregnancy is one in which the fertilized ovum implants in some site other than the uterine cavity. Ectopic pregnancy remains an important cause of maternal death in the UK and worldwide.[1,2] According to the latest UK Confidential Enquiry report, there were 10 maternal deaths resulting from ectopic pregnancy between 2003–2005.[1]

Around a third of tubal pregnancies occur in women with current or previous evidence of tubal damage due to surgery or infection, with increasing episodes of pelvic inflammatory disease significantly increasing risk. Other risk factors:

- Smoking.
- Current or previous use of an intrauterine contraceptive device: whether levonorgestrel-based or conventional.
- Current use of a progesterone based contraceptive.
- Sterilization.
- Assisted reproductive techniques roughly double the risk of ectopic pregnancy.[3]

### Epidemiology

- 1% of recognized pregnancies in the UK, but around 2% in the USA.
- Around 93% of ectopic pregnancies are tubal.

### Clinical features and non-imaging investigations

The clinical features of ectopic pregnancy are bleeding and abdominal pain following amenorrhoea. However, many women are asymptomatic and some may deny that they may be pregnant, as an episode of vaginal bleeding may be erroneously considered to be menstruation. *There is considerable overlap between the symptoms of ectopic pregnancy and those of miscarriage.* Some women may present with an episode of syncope and vaginal bleeding. Symptoms and clinical signs particularly suspicious for ectopic pregnancy are:

- Shoulder tip pain
- An acute abdomen with rebound tenderness and guarding
- Vaginal examination may elicit cervical excitation, adnexal tenderness or an adnexal mass.

A urine pregnancy test will almost always be positive. Serum will normally be taken and hCG levels (and progesterone in some units) will be quantified. Serum hCG levels aids assessment of the likelihood of ectopic pregnancy if an intrauterine pregnancy cannot be visualized on ultrasound and help to decide if medical, surgical or even expectant management is appropriate.[2] In general, an intrauterine gestation is usually visible on transvaginal ultrasound when serum $\beta$-hCG concentration has reached 1500IU/L–2000IU/L ('the discriminatory zone').[3] Highly skilled operators may be able to identify a pregnancy sac at lower serum hCG levels than this. An approximate corresponding threshold for transabdominal US is 6500IU/L.[3] However, in multiple pregnancies, serum $\beta$-hCG levels are higher than for singleton pregnancies for a given gestational age, and this should also be considered.

## Imaging

### US

*Protocol*

Perform a pelvic survey with a curvilinear abdominal (3–5MHz) probe. If the bladder is empty, identifying the uterus (especially if retroverted) and adnexal structures may be difficult. Transvaginal US (7–8MHz) is recommended. Identify the uterus and cervix in a sagittal plane and sweep laterally in both directions. Check for a gestation sac, free fluid in the pelvis, and adnexal pathology.

*Findings*

- Appearances of ectopic pregnancy are variable on TVUS.[4] The 'classical' findings are of an empty uterus with a hyperechoic ring around the gestation sac in the adnexal region. However, most ectopic pregnancies appear as an inhomogenous mass or 'blob' next to the ovary, with no sign of a sac or embryo. Any mass should be measured, as should the presence of any fetal heart activity.
- An intrauterine 'pseudosac' will often be seen and should not be confused with an early gestation sac. The absence of an echogenic rim of chorionic tissue helps to distinguish the pseudosac from a true gestation sac.
- Free fluid is seen within the pouch of Douglas in around 20–25% of ectopic pregnancies, but is non-specific as it may also be seen following rupture of a corpus luteum cyst. The corpus luteum will be on the same side as the ectopic in 70–85% of cases.[4]
- The possibility of rarer sites of ectopic pregnancy should be considered, including interstitial (cornual) tubal pregnancy (2% of ectopics), cervical pregnancy (0.2% of ectopics), Caesarean scar and ovarian pregnancy (<1% ectopics).[4] Coexisting intrauterine and ectopic pregnancies may also occur ('heterotopic pregnancy'), especially following IVF.
- No pregnancy may be seen—a 'pregnancy of unknown location' or PUL.[4]

## Differential diagnosis

- Miscarriage.
- Intrauterine pregnancy with coexistent adnexal or pelvic pathology.

## Management

- Laparoscopic surgery (salpingectomy or salpingostomy) is the commonest treatment modality.
- Medical treatment (e.g. with systemic methotrexate) or even conservative treatment.
- Laparotomy is still appropriate for cases with haemodynamic instability.
- Anti-D should be given to Rhesus negative women after treatment.

## Further reading

**1.** Lewis, G (ed.) (2007) *Saving mother's lives: reviewing maternal deaths to make motherhood safer 2003–2005. The Seventh Report on Confidential Enquiries into Maternal Deaths in the United Kingdom.* London: CEMACH. http://www.cemach.org.uk.

**2.** RCOG (2004) *The Management of Tubal Pregnancy.* Greentop Guideline 21, available at http://www.rcog.org.uk/resources/Public/pdf/management_tubal_pregnancy210pdf.

**3.** Farquhar CM (2005) Ectopic pregnancy. *Lancet* **366**: 583–91.

**4.** Bourne T and Condous G (2006) *Handbook of Early Pregnancy Care.* Abingdon: Informa Healthcare.

# ① ⑦ **Bleeding in late pregnancy**

### Definition and aetiology

Vaginal bleeding from 24 week gestations until delivery of the fetus is defined as antepartum haemorrhage. Bleeding before this point has historically been considered 'threatened miscarriage'. Inevitably there is considerable overlap between the aetiology and management of these conditions.

Bleeding in the 3rd trimester of pregnancy—after 24 weeks gestation—may be due to:
- retroplacental bleeding/partial separation of a normally sited placenta ('abruption')
- partial separation of a low-lying placenta ('placenta praevia', which may be morbidly adherent 'placenta accreta')
- bleeding from cervical or vaginal lesions
- bleeding from abnormally sited fetal vessels ('vasa praevia')

### Epidemiology

Very common problem, affects 2–5% of pregnancies. Minor abruptions may only be diagnosed after delivery. Placenta praevia affects approximately 0.3–0.5% of pregnancies at term, but is more common pre-term. The 2nd trimester incidence of a placenta praevia varies from 1.1% (if a transvaginal US approach is used) to 15–20% (if a transabdominal approach is used).[1] Vasa praevia has an incidence of approximately 1:2500 pregnancies.[1] The incidence of placenta accreta has been estimated at between 1:2510 and 1:533 pregnancies,[1] but is probably becoming more common as the Caesarean section rate increases in many hospitals.

### Clinical features

- Vaginal bleeding may be variable from a streak of blood to massive haemorrhage and hypovolemic shock.
- Bleeding may be accompanied by pain (usually cramping, like menstrual pain, or backache), and/or uterine activity. It may have been precipitated, e.g. by sexual intercourse, or unprovoked. The association of pain suggests an intrauterine bleed and is more typical of abruption. Pain is less common with bleeds due to placenta praevia, as the blood may leave the uterus via the cervix without uterine irritation.
- There may be uterine tenderness, signs of fetal compromise, or even fetal death.
- Vasa praevia may be suspected when there is rupture of the membranes is accompanied by accompanied by vaginal bleeding and signs of fetal distress and/or death.

Speculum examination may be performed to assess the quantity of bleeding and to assess for local causes, e.g. cervical pathology, when placenta praevia has been excluded, and to determine if there is cervical dilatation.

### Imaging

*The main role of imaging is to confirm placental site, and to determine fetal viability.*

- Most women will have had placental site determined at their 18–23 week scan.
- US is unreliable in the making the diagnosis of placental abruption.
- US is the investigation of choice in the diagnosis of placental praevia.
- US will also be helpful in the assessment of fetal growth and well-being, especially in women who present with recurrent antepartum haemorrhage attributed to minor abruptions.
- MRI has been reported to be useful in the assessment of placenta accreta, that is an abnormally invasive placenta.

## US
### Protocol
Abdominal or pelvic US with curvilinear probe (3–5MHz adults). Identify the lower uterine segment, which is covered anteriorly by the bladder. For posterior placentae, it may be necessary to perform transvaginal US to assess the relationship between the leading edge of the placenta and the internal cervical os, due to acoustic shadowing from the fetal skull in the 3rd trimester. Transvaginal US is superior to transabdominal US in the assessment of placenta praevia.[1]

### Findings
- In a major placenta praevia, the leading edge of the placenta encroaches on or covers the internal cervical os.
- In a minor placenta praevia, the leading edge of the placenta encroaches into the lower segment.
- It is helpful for clinicians to know the distance of the leading placental edge from the internal os and the relative position of the presenting part in relation to the placental edge and/or the internal cervical os. This measurement should be normally be based on a TV assessment.[1,2]
- Placenta accreta is most likely in the context of anterior placenta praevia in a woman who has had previous Caesarean section. Greyscale, power and colour flow Doppler may all be of value in the diagnosis of abnormally adherent placenta. The presence of irregularly shaped placental lacunae, thinning of the myometrium in the placental implantation site, and apparent protrusion of the placenta into the bladder are among the features suggestive of placenta accreta.[1]
- Vasa praevia may be suspected by the identification of linear echolucent structures overlying the cervix on greyscale. Power or colour Doppler may demonstrate blood flow within these vessels. Pulsed Doppler of these structures may demonstrate the typical waveforms of the fetal umbilical artery or vein.[1]

## MRI
MRI has been used in the assessment of suspected placenta accreta; it is unlikely to be appropriate in the acute situation. The interested reader should refer to references 1 and 2 below for further details.

## Management

Management depends on the underlying cause.

- For major placenta praevia, delivery will be by Caesarean section at 38 weeks or sooner if mandated by maternal or fetal condition. For minor degrees of placenta praevia, a vaginal delivery may be feasible but facilities should be available for Caesarean section and blood transfusion in the event of significant intrapartum haemorrhage. If there is placenta accreta, hysterectomy or other surgical procedures (or embolization of uterine vessels) may be necessary to prevent or control life threatening haemorrhage.[1,2]

- In placental abruption, the condition of the fetus will determine whether vaginal delivery is appropriate. Labour may be rapid with intrapartum abruption but fetal compromise may ensue before full dilatation is reached.
- For anything more than a trivial bleed, IV access should be established, and blood sent for FBC, clotting and group and save serum/cross-match.
- If immediate delivery is not anticipated, the mother should receive antenatal steroids if preterm delivery is likely.
- Rhesus negative women should receive anti-D prophylaxis unless the fetus is known to be Rhesus negative also.

**Further reading**
1. Oyelese Y and Smulian JC (2006) Placenta previa, placenta accreta, and vasa previa. *Obstet Gynecol* **107(4)**; 927–41.

2. RCOG (2005) *Placenta Previa and Placenta Praevia Accreta: Diagnosis and Management.* Greentop Guideline 27, available at http://www.rcog.org.uk/resources/Public/pdf/placenta_previa_accreta.pdf.

# ☼ ① Post-partum haemorrhage (PPH)

### Definition and aetiology

Bleeding from the genital tract after delivery of more than 500ml. It occurs in around 5–10% of deliveries in the UK and is responsible for around 11% (around 140,000) of maternal deaths worldwide.[1] Unfortunately, the estimation of blood loss at both vaginal and Caesarean deliveries is rather subjective and frequently underestimated. The possibility of occult bleeding should be considered.

- **Primary PPH :** >500ml blood loss (or any amount causing haemodynamic disturbance) within 24hrs of delivery.
- **Secondary PPH:** >500ml after 24hrs but within 6 weeks of delivery.
- **Massive obstetric PPH:** >1500ml may be life-threatening and requires rapid action to prevent death.

Causes are the '4 Ts':

- Tone: uterine atony is the commonest cause
- Trauma: to cervix, vagina, perineum, uterus and tears into the broad ligament
- Tissue: retained placenta and placental fragments
- Thrombin: coagulopathy following massive haemorrhage, pre-eclampsia, abruption, amniotic fluid embolism and sepsis. Pre-existing maternal bleeding disorder (e.g. Von Willebrand's disease, haemophilia carrier status) may also contribute to haemorrhage.[2]

Antenatal Risk factors—according to NICE Guidelines:[3]

- Previous retained placenta or PPH
- Maternal haemoglobin <8.5g/dl prior to labour
- Body mass index >35 kg/m$^2$
- Grand multiparity (parity 4 or more)
- Antepartum haemorrhage (especially abruption and placenta previa)
- Overdistention of the uterus (e.g. multiple pregnancy/polyhydramnios)
- Anatomical uterine abnormalities
- Maternal age of 35yrs or older

Intrapartum risk factors—according to NICE Guidelines[3]

- Operative delivery
- Induction of labour
- Prolonged 1st, 2nd or 3rd stage of labour
- Oxytocin use
- Precipitate labour

### Epidemiology

Very common problem, affects 5–10% of pregnancies.

### Clinical features

Vaginal bleeding may be variable from a streak of blood to massive haemorrhage and hypovolemic shock. Bleeding may be concealed: there may be intra-abdominal bleeding, or paravaginal in the cases of perineal haematoma.

## Imaging

Imaging usually has a limited role in the assessment of post-partum haemorrhage, as the majority of these have a clinically apparent cause. Atonic PPH, the commonest cause, is diagnosed clinically by assessment/palpation of uterine tone. Ultrasound may be used acutely in the labour ward setting if the placenta is suspected to be incomplete at delivery, or following presentation with secondary PPH, a leading cause for which is retained placental fragments. It may also be helpful in the diagnosis of suspected intra-abdominal bleeding.

### US

*Protocol*

Abdominal with curvilinear probe (3–5MHz adults). Visualize the uterus, and sweep through the uterus in all planes to look for any retained placental fragments. Frequently there will be blood clot within the cavity presenting as mixed echogenicities. Following Caesarean delivery, when intra-abdominal bleeding may be suspected, look for free fluid in the pelvis, and evidence of haematoma in the utero-vesical pouch, and the broad ligament.

### Management

- Management depends on the underlying cause.
- For acute post-partum haemorrhage, treatment of uterine atony includes aggressive fluid resuscitation, and administration of oxytocic agents such as oxytocin, ergometrine, carboprost and misoprostol.
- Retained placental tissue must normally be removed, and perineal, vaginal and cervical trauma repaired, which may require examination under spinal or general anaesthesia.
- For secondary PPH, conservative management, with prophylatic antibiotics, is often appropriate.
- Surgical procedures including uterine compression sutures, ligation of the uterine or internal iliac arteries, and hysterectomy may also be necessary.
- Occasionally, interventional radiology (arterial embolization) may be of assistance in controlling persistent bleeding despite the above.

### Further reading

**1.** CEMACH (2007) *Saving Mothers' Lives: Confidential Inquiry into Maternal and Child Health, 7th Report.* CEMACH, London.

**2.** Lee CA, Chi C, Pavord SR *et al.* (2006) The obstetric and gynaecological management of women with inherited bleeding disorders: review with guidelines produced by a task force of UK Heamophilia Centre Doctors' Organization. *Haemophilia* **12**; 301–36.

**3.** NICE (2007) *Intrapartum Care.* NICE Clinical Guideline 55, available at http://www.nice.org.uk.

# Breast emergencies

The usual focus of breast radiology is either the screening of asymptomatic women or evaluation of patients with breast symptoms, most commonly a lump, for possible carcinoma. Emergencies affecting the breast that require radiological input are rare but they do occur, and correct identification along with rapid appropriate management will minimise associated morbidity.

## Imaging

- In the emergency setting, most assessment will be clinical followed by ultrasound in the light of a relevant history.
- Occasionally vascular intervention may be required to embolize a bleeding vessel.
- There are few emergency indications for mammography or MRI.
- The breasts are frequently imaged during CT examinations and incidental findings are relatively common (📖 p. 335).

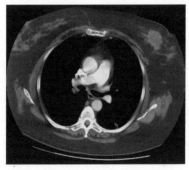

**Fig. 12.6** Incidental finding of a breast cancer on chest CT: there is an irregular area of increased attenuation within the left breast. Also note the metastasis in the left lung.

## US

- The main role of ultrasound is to determine the presence and extent of any collection. An assessment of the need for drainage can be made and this can then be performed, under image guidance if necessary (📖 p. 335).
- Typically collections contain pus (abscesses) or blood (haematomas).
- The ultrasound appearance is variable depending on the relative amount of fluid and solid components. The liquefied centre of a collection may be aspirated, the inflammatory surrounding tissue cannot.
- Use the highest frequency probe that gives adequate penetration to the lesion. In patients with large breasts or an extensive abnormality, scan the area with a lower frequency probe first to ensure that there is not a more extensive deeper collection that cannot be appreciated using the high-frequency probe.

- Usually there will be some areas of fluid which appear as anechoic regions with posterior acoustic enhancement.
- Often there is surrounding inflamed tissue which typically appears hypervascular on Doppler imaging.
- Less commonly, assessment of breast implant rupture can be made.

# Breast abscess

### Aetiology

May develop as a complication to mastitis (particularly in lactating women), post biopsy/operation or as a result of infection around a pre existing lesion.

### Clinical features

- Most commonly occur in central/subareolar area.
- Clinical features: fever, pain, local tenderness with erythema of skin, increased inflammatory markers and white cell count.

### Imaging

#### US

Are often multi loculated hence one or more areas of low reflectivity are visible on ultrasound with hyper vascular surrounding inflammatory tissue giving a high signal on Doppler imaging.

### Management

- Aspiration alone may be effective, particularly for smaller (<3cm) unilocule lesions.
- The alternative is to leave an indwelling drain *in situ* or perform a surgical washout.
- Discussion with senior radiologists/ breast surgeons is recommended as local practice varies.

# Breast haematoma

## Aetiology

- Often post-traumatic (usually blunt injury such as a blow or seat belt injury), post biopsy or post operative. Rarely carcinoma may present as haematoma.
- More common in patients with abnormal clotting (e.g. anticoagulants, recent thrombolysis or haematological disease.) Particularly in these patients, breast haematoma may be spontaneous.

## Imaging

### US

- Variable appearance on US; usually they are of mixed echogenicity with some fluid components of low reflectivity though there is a spectrum of appearances ranging from an almost cystic to an almost solid-looking lesion. There may be some increased flow on Doppler due to surrounding inflammation although usually less than surrounding an abscess.
- Rarely, active bleeding will be visible on Doppler imaging. (e.g. false aneurysm)

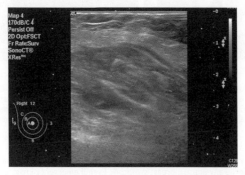

Fig. 12.7  US image demonstrating the variable appearance of a breast haematoma.

## Management

- The need for intervention will depend on the size and overlying skin.
  - Intervention is required if the skin becomes taught or thinned because gangrene due to pressure necrosis is a risk if the pressure is not relieved.
- Small haematomas may usually be managed conservatively with analgesia and a supportive bra.

# Other breast conditions

### Assessment of suspected ruptured breast implant

- May be spontaneous or following trauma (e.g. seatbelt injury)
- Implant rupture may be intra- or extra-capsular (a fibrous capsule is formed around the implant over time and this may contain a rupture).
- An implant may have a double lumen and care is needed not to mis-diagnose a double border as a rupture.
- Extra-capsular rupture should be suspected if a highly reflective area of silicone extrudes from the implant causing acoustic shadowing: *snowstorm*. However, the extruded material may occasionally also mimic a cyst and be close to anechoic.
- Intra-capsular rupture may appear as a series of parallel straight lines: the *stepladder sign*.
- Implant rupture may be confirmed on MRI.

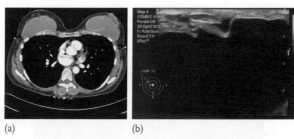

(a)                                    (b)

**Fig. 12.8** Breast implant rupture. (a) Intracapsular rupture demonstrated on CT. There is a linear density within the left implant which is a fold of the ruptured shell (Analogous to the linguine sign on MRI), (b) Ultrasound image of an intracapsular rupture. The outer rim of the breast implant is irregular with parallel echogenic lines.

### Breast carcinoma

- Very rarely presents as a breast emergency although a carcinoma may underlie any unusual breast symptom. Even if emergency imaging is not indicated, follow-up should be recommended.

### Fat necrosis

- Tends to present some time after trauma rather than as an emergency and the history of trauma may be occult.
- Seen as a complication is approximately 0.5% breast biopsies.
- Aspiration yields yellowish fatty fluid

## Breasts on CT

- CT is not usually the chosen modality for breast imaging but abnormalities may be apparent, either in patients in whom breast pathology has already been diagnosed or as an incidental finding.
- Further evaluation with more appropriate modalities should be arranged if there is any suspicion of an abnormality.
- Most often an abnormality will be a soft tissue mass with or without lymphadenopathy but collections, abnormal calcification, lymphatic congestion or implant rupture may also be visible.
- In the emergency setting, ultrasound would be appropriate if there is suspicion of haematoma, abscess or implant rupture. Mammography should be considered if there is suspicion of malignancy.

## Other relevant chapters/sections

- Sedation and analgesia ☐ p. 32.
- Embolization/coiling of bleeding vessels ☐ p. 384.

---

### How to drain a superficial collection under ultrasound

- Either 'no touch' technique after marking spot or direct guidance.
- Use local anaesthetic (e.g. 1% lidocaine) if making multiple passes, using a wide-bore needle or siting a drain.
- 1. 'No touch' technique:
  - Perform diagnostic scan, mark suitable spot, measure depth and note angle of approach. (Easiest if approach is made at 90° to skin.)
  - Clean the site and then puncture without rescanning or touching the skin. Hold skin taught with other hand.
  - Advance needle with syringe attached along pre-judged line, while aspirating continuously until fluid is obtained.
  - Drain collection to dryness.
- 2. Direct guidance (scanning with needle in continuous view):
  - This is a better technique if the collection is not easy to reach or is small. It may also be used if target is close to important structures, although this is uncommon in the breast.
  - Clean the skin. Sterilize the probe or use a sterile probe cover.
  - Begin with the target lesion in vision and the needle adjacent to one end of the US probe. Note the depth and distance required to gauge the approximate angle required.
  - Advance the needle in the plane of the ultrasound beam towards the target site/depth watching the *tip* of the needle.
  - Be careful to keep the needle in the plane of the beam. Direct observation of the probe and needle is helpful. Gentle rocking of the probe perpendicular to the track of the needle can help to ensure that the tip remains visible.
  - If the needle is not on target then pull back and start again from near the surface. Do not try to change the angle of the track when already deep in the soft tissues as the superficial tissue will have a splinting effect and prevent any change being transmitted to the needle tip.

## Further reading

**1.** Hook GW and Ikeda DM (1999) Treatment of breast abscesses with US-guided percutaneous needle drainage without indwelling catheter placement. *Radiology* **213**; 579–82.

**2.** Ulitzsch D, Nyman MKG and Carlson RA (2004) Breast abscess in lactating women: US-guided treatment. *Radiology* **232**; 904–9.

**3.** Gatta G, Pinto S, Romano A *et al.* (2007) Clinical, mammographic and ultrasonographic features of blunt breast trauma. *European Journal of Radiology* **59(3)**; 327–30.

# Paediatrics

Howard Portess
Ash Chakraborty

# ⊙ **Intussusception**

The invagination of one segment of the bowel (intussusceptum) into the lumen of the distal portion of the same loop of bowel·(intussuscipiens). The commonest type is ileocolic (95%) followed by ileoileal (4%) and colocolic.

## Aetiology
- Idiopathic (95%): although the cause is unclear, it frequently follows viral gastroenteritis and is possibly due to mucosal oedema and lymphoid hyperplasia.
- Meckel's diverticulum: commonest cause of ileoileal intussusception.
- Duplication cysts.
- Lymphoma.
- Polyps.
- Henoch–Schönlein purpura.

## Clinical features
Typically occurs between 3 months and 3 years of age and symptoms include:
- Sudden onset of colicky abdominal pain.
- Abdominal distension.
- 'Redcurrant jelly' stools due to sloughed mucus and blood.
- Palpable abdominal mass (60%): commonly in the right upper quadrant.

## Imaging
### Radiographs
*Findings*
- Gasless abdomen.
- Soft tissue mass with concentric circular lucencies of entrapped mesenteric fat.
- If the distal bowel is gas filled, the lead point of the intussusception can be seen as a rounded mass ('meniscus sign').

### Ultrasound
*Protocol*
First interrogate with a 6–10MHz curvilinear probe, dependent on patient size (the smaller the patient the higher frequency the probe). Perform a general abdominal and pelvic ultrasound examination of the solid organs and bowel. Next use a 5–10MHz linear probe, dependent on patient size, scanning each quadrant of the abdomen to assess the bowel. Perform Doppler interrogation of the intussusception which is typically located in the right upper quadrant.

*Findings*
- 'Doughnut sign' (Fig. 13.1a).
- 'Pseudokidney sign': (Fig. 13.1b).
- Features which increase the likelihood that reduction will fail:
  - No Doppler flow present due to possible ischaemia and necrosis.
  - Fluid trapped in layers of the intussusception.
  - Duration of symptoms is >48 hrs.

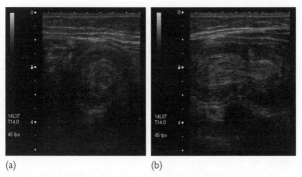

(a)                                    (b)

**Fig. 13.1** (a) Transverse image shows a central low echogenicity intussusceptum surrounded by echogenic mesentery and the low echogenicity intussuscipiens. (b) Oblique image shows hypoehoic layers of bowel wall surrounding the central echogenic mesenteric fat.

## Management

The favoured treatment is radiological air enema reduction. Barium can be used but increases difficulty of the surgical laparotomy if the reduction fails; also the risk of barium peritonitis if the bowel perforates, has led to this technique becoming rarely used. Radiological reduction should be performed by a senior radiologist with adequate training and ongoing experience and when there is suitable paediatric surgical and anaesthetic support. If these are not available transfer to a specialist unit should be arranged.

### Patient preparation
- NG tube.
- IV access and fluid bolus prior to the procedure.
- IV antibiotics.

### Parental consent
- Aim: to relieve the obstruction.
- Risks: failure of reduction, perforation and recurrence of the intussusception. Failure and perforation rates vary between institutions and the recurrence rate is generally 10%.
- They should also consent to a laparotomy if perforation occurs.
- Intussusception reduction is distressing for both the child and the parents and it may be better for the parents not to be present during the reduction.

### Equipment and assistants
- Oxygen saturation monitor.
- Paediatric resuscitation trolley.
- Oxygen and suction.
- 12 G needle or cannula (for emergency decompression: see below).
- 24–26 Fr Foley catheter.

- Intussusception reduction device: hand or mechanical pump with pressure monitor and safety pressure release valve or water column manometer system.
- Assistants to help hold the child with appropriate lead shielding.
- Senior experienced nurse to help hold and to monitor oxygen saturations.
- Senior member of surgical team capable of taking the patient directly to theatre should the bowel perforate.
- At least one person trained in paediatric life support.

*Protocol*

Lay the patient supine on the screening table and insert the catheter into the rectum and firmly tape in place. Take a control image of sufficient quality (either a fluoroscopic image or abdominal radiograph) to exclude free gas due to perforation.

One assistant squeezes the patient's buttocks to make a seal as air is pumped into the rectum to an initial maximum pressure of 80mmHg. Using intermittent screening follow the progress of the reduction and regularly store fluoroscopic images during the procedure. Maintain pressure for 3min. Successful reduction is defined as reflux of gas into the small bowel. If unsuccessful, release the pressure and rest for 3min. Make a second 3min attempt at 100mmHg. If still unsuccessful, rest for 3min and make a third attempt at 120mmHg ('Rule of 3s').

It is common to reduce to the ileocaecal valve but have no reflux into the small bowel. A repeat attempt after 2–3hrs may be successful by allowing oedema of the valve to reduce. If there is still a significant intussusceptum within the colon, then surgery is indicated.

## Complications of reduction

- Respiratory compromise. Gaseous distension of the bowel splints the diaphragm. Stop the reduction and release the pressure if the nurse tells you they are concerned about the patient and the oxygen saturations are low.
- Perforation. Watch for the development of Riglers' sign or subdiaphragmatic air. *If there is any doubt then stop the reduction and take an exposure (abdominal radiograph).* The most serious form of free air in the abdomen is a tension pneumoperitoneum. This blocks venous return from the lower body and splints the diaphragm leading to rapid cardiorespiratory collapse and death. Rapid decompression by insertion of a needle or cannula into the midline below the umbilicus is required to decompress the tension pneumoperitoneum.

## Further reading

**1.** AT Byrne (2005) The imaging of intussusception. *Clinical Radiology* **60**; 39–46.

# ① Small bowel malrotation and volvulus

The normal small bowel mesentery extends from the duodenojejunal flexure in the left upper quadrant to the ileocaecal valve in the right lower quadrant. Failure to complete normal gut rotation (malrotation) *in utero* leads to a shortening of this mesentery which reduces small bowel stability and increases the likelihood of it twisting on its own mesentery (volvulus). This can lead to bowel obstruction, ischaemia and necrosis.

## Clinical features

- 80% in first week of life and most have volvulus at presentation.
  Symptoms include:
  - Bilious vomiting.
  - Abdominal pain and distension.
- 20% present at any age with vague symptoms due to intermittent volvulus.

## Imaging

### *Upper GI contrast study*

An upper GI contrast study is the investigation of choice for malrotation.

*Protocol*

Contrast media can be given orally or via an NG tube. In outpatients, use barium but if acutely unwell use a water-soluble agent, e.g. Iopamidol 200.

Place the patient on their right side on the screening table. Fill the antrum of the stomach with a small amount of contrast and wait for the stomach to empty with intermittent screening. If the stomach is completely full the duodenojejunal flexure may be obscured and possibly displaced.

The contrast medium moves posteriorly through the first part of the duodenum and inferiorly and parallel to the spine through the second part. When the contrast starts to move superiorly as it enters the fourth part of the duodenum turn the patient supine ensuring their shoulders and hips are flat on the table (Fig. 13.2). Screen the right upper quadrant and include the left lung base and lower mediastinum to demonstrate any rotation of the patient. The duodenojejunal flexure is the point at which the ascending fourth part of the duodenum turns laterally or inferiorly to become the jejunum.

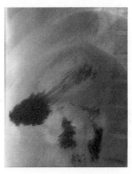

**Fig. 13.2** Lateral view showing contrast arriving in the fourth part of the duodenum.

*Findings*

The flexure should lie to the left of the left pedicle of L2 which is the same level as the first part of the duodenum (Fig. 13.3). If it is lower or more to the right than this there is malrotation.

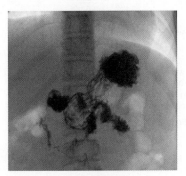

**Fig. 13.3** Normal position of the duodenojejunal flexure.

Continue to follow the contrast into the proximal loops of jejunum and look for the corkscrew appearance of a volvulus. If the volvulus is tight then there is a tapering beak termination to the contrast medium.

*US*

Reversal of the normal relationship of the superior mesenteric artery and vein is unreliable and a normal appearance does not exclude malrotation.

### Management

If malrotation alone is found then urgent fixation of the bowel is indicated to prevent future volvulus. However, if volvulus is present at the time of the study then emergency surgery is required to relieve the obstruction and prevent ischaemic damage and the appropriate team should be contacted urgently.

### Differential diagnosis

- Duodenal atresia.
- Duodenal web.
- Pyloric stenosis.
- Ladd's bands.
- Reflux.

### Further reading

**1.** Strouse PJ (2004) Disorders of intestinal rotation and fixation ('malrotation'). *Pediatr Radiol* **34**; 837–51.

**2.** Ashley LM (2001) A normal sonogram does not exclude malrotation. *Pediatr Radiol* **31**; 354–6.

**3.** Sizemore AW (2008) Diagnostic performance of the upper gastrointestinal series in the evaluation of children with clinically suspected malrotation. *Pediatr Radiol* **38**; 518–28.

# ① ⑦ **Bowel obstruction**

In neonates and babies the appearance of large and small bowel on plain films is very similar, therefore obstruction is usually divided into high and low obstruction.

## Aetiology of paediatric bowel obstruction

### High obstruction
- Duodenal atresia.
- Duodenal web.
- SMA syndrome.
- Malrotation and volvulus (see 📖 p 342).
- Pyloric stenosis (see 📖 p 360).

### Low obstruction
- Ileal atresia.
- Meconium ileus.
- Meconium plug syndrome.
- Hirschprung's disease.

## Imaging
### Radiographs
*Findings*
- High obstruction:
  - Few dilated gas-filled loops of bowel.
  - Further investigation required with an upper GI contrast study.
- Low obstruction:
  - Many dilated loops of gas-filled bowel.
  - Further investigation required with a contrast enema.

# High obstruction

## Duodenal atresia

Failure of recanalisation of the second part of the duodenum usually just distal to the Ampulla of Vater.

### Clinical features

- May have antenatal diagnosis (polyhydramnios and dilated stomach).
- Usually diagnosed in the first 24hrs of life.
- Bilious vomiting.
- Failure to pass meconium.

### Imaging

### *Radiographs: AXR*

*Findings*

Double bubble: gas-filled dilated stomach and first part of duodenum. No gas elsewhere in the abdomen. Plain film is diagnostic and no further investigation is necessary.

There is a rare situation of interconnected main and accessory pancreatic ducts where one inserts proximal and one distal to the obstruction which allows a small amount of gas to pass beyond the obstruction.

## Duodenal web

Partial recanalization of duodenum leaving a web with a small aperture in the second part of the duodenum.

### Clinical features

- Can be any age with earlier presentation in those with a smaller aperture.
- Bilious vomiting.
- Poor weight gain.
- Failure to thrive.

### *Radiographs: AXR*

*Findings*

- Often normal.
- May show dilated stomach and proximal duodenum with variable amount of gas elsewhere in abdomen.

### *Upper GI contrast study*

*Protocol*

Perform a standard paediatric upper GI study (see malrotation 📖 p. 342).

*Findings*

A large-volume stomach which often empties slowly and a dilated duodenum with pooling of contrast medium. The column of contrast medium has a straight or convex leading edge and there are many non-propulsive peristalsis waves. A narrow jet of contrast may be seen to squirt forwards into a normal calibre distal duodenal segment. In the more chronic situation the web stretches to form a 'windsock' shape.

# Superior mesenteric artery syndrome

Compression of the third part of the duodenum by the superior mesenteric artery (SMA) against the aorta.

## Aetiology

Predisposing factors include:
- Thin constitution.
- Rapid weight loss.
- Excessive lumbar lordosis.
- Cerebral palsy.
- Spinal jacket.

## Clinical features
- Usually in older children and adolescents.
- Intermittent vomiting.
- Abdominal pain after eating.
- Poor weight gain/weight loss.

## Imaging

### Radiographs: AXR

*Findings*

Usually normal or dilated stomach.

### Upper GI contrast study

*Protocol*

Perform a standard paediatric upper GI study (📖 Malrotation and volvulus p. 342).

*Findings*

The appearance is similar to a duodenal web. However, the leading edge of the column of contrast is in the midline and straight. Very little contrast passes the midline whilst the patient is supine, but turning the patient prone allows the SMA to be displaced anteriorly which reduces the compression, allowing contrast medium to pass into the distal duodenum which is of normal calibre.

# Low obstruction

## Ileal atresia

An ischaemic event *in utero* leads to stricture formation and obstruction comonest in the distal ileum.

**Clinical features**
- Presents in first 24hrs of life.
- Failure to pass meconium.
- Abdominal distension.
- Bilious vomiting.

### Imaging
### Radiographs: AXR
*Findings*
Multiple dilated loops of bowel.

### Contrast enema
*Patient preparation*
Ensure the patient has an NG tube and IV access.

*Protocol*
Use low osmolar water-soluble contrast medium e.g. Iopamidol 150–200 to reduce the risk of large volume fluid shift into the bowel. Higher concentration contrast can be diluted with water. Insert an 8–12 Fr (depending on patient size) Foley catheter into the rectum and tape in position. Put the patient on their left side. Squeeze the buttocks to make a seal and inject the contrast slowly storing images of the rectum and sigmoid colon. Place the patient supine and continue to inject contrast medium. Using intermittent screening store fluoroscopic images of the colon. Aim to fill the entire colon and image contrast medium refluxing into the terminal ileum.

*Findings*
Total colonic microcolon with few filling defects. The contrast medium may distend the rectum. Contrast medium refluxes into the terminal ileum but does not reach any dilated bowel. When the catheter is removed clear fluid (contrast medium) is expelled.

## Meconium ileus

Thick inspissated meconium causes a mechanical obstruction. Commonly associated with cystic fibrosis.

**Clinical features**
- Often diagnosed antenatally because of echogenic bowel on US.
- Presents in first 24hrs of life.
- Failure to pass meconium.
- Abdominal distension.

## Imaging
### Radiographs: AXR
*Findings*
- Multiple dilated loops of bowel.
- Mottled bowel in right lower quadrant due to air mixed with meconium.

### Contrast enema
*Protocol*
Perform a standard paediatric contrast enema (📖 Ileal atresia p. 348).

The use of gastrografin in this situation is controversial. Traditionally gastrografin was used for two reasons: it has high osmolarity and causes a fluid shift into the lumen of the bowel which loosens and flushes out the meconium; secondly gastrografin contains Tween-80, a soap-like substance which lubricates the bowel, emulsifies the meconium and aids passage. However, gastrografin causes massive fluid shift into the bowel and unless there is careful observation and IV fluid replacement, the patient can suffer from cardiovascular collapse. Water-soluble contrast media such as Iopamidol is often effective. Most departments will have a local policy about the use of gastrografin. *If there is any doubt about the use of gastrografin it should be avoided, as the mechanical effect of the enema may be sufficient.*

*Findings*
A microcolon with a few filling defects. Differentiate this from ileal atresia by refluxing contrast into dilated small bowel containing one or more filling defects. The expelled contrast is commonly stained green and may contain meconium pellets (Fig. 13.4).

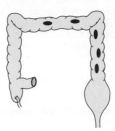

**Fig. 13.4** Total colonic microcolon with a few filling defects.

## Management
If no meconium is passed and the abdomen remains distended then surgery is required. If there is clinical improvement but the patient remains obstructed a repeat enema may be of benefit.

# Meconium plug syndrome

Functional obstruction of bowel due imaturity of the ganglion cells innervating the colon.

## Clinical features
- Presents in first 24hrs of life.
- Failure to pass meconium.
- Abdominal distension.

## Imaging
### Radiographs: AXR
*Findings*
Multiple dilated loops of bowel.

### Contrast enema
*Protocol*
Perform a standard paediatric contrast enema (📖 Ileal atresia p. 348).
   As with meconium ileus, the choice of contrast is controversial.

*Findings*
There are multiple meconium plugs seen within the colon. The colon is often of normal or increased calibre throughout. If the left colon is narrowed with a transition to dilated colon at the splenic flexure, it can be impossible to differentiate from Hirschsprung's disease.

# Hirschsprung's disease

Hirschsprung's disease or myenteric plexus aganglionosis always involves the anus and internal sphincter and extends proximally by a variable distance. This leads to a failure of muscle relaxation in the abnormal region and consequent proximal dilatation. Distribution:
- 75% rectosigmoid or short segment disease.
- 15–20% long segment disease.
- 5–10% total colonic disease.
- Very short segment disease is very rare.

## Clinical features
- Usually presents in first week of life but can appear at any age.
- Failure to pass meconium.
- Abdominal distension.
- Chronic constipation.

## Imaging
### Radiographs: AXR
*Findings*
Multiple dilated loops of bowel with paucity of rectal gas.

### Contrast enema
This starts with a more focused look at the rectum and sigmoid colon. An enema or a PR examination in the 24hrs prior to the study can dilate the rectum leading to a false negative result. If the patient is well and the

clinical requirement is to exclude Hirschprung's disease then the enema should be delayed. If the patient is unwell and the clinical requirement is for a therapeutic effect then proceed with the enema.

*Protocol*

Place the patient on their left side and insert a small 8–10 Fr Foley catheter into the rectum with the hole lying just above the junction of the rectum and the anal canal. Start with full-strength water-soluble contrast (e.g. Iopamidol 300) and slowly inject a small amount whilst screening and store these early fluoroscopic images. Aim to fill the lumen of the rectum and sigmoid colon without artificially dilating it. If the sigmoid colon is not dilated continue the procedure with half-strength contrast and complete the enema as above.

*Findings*

The hallmark of Hirschsprung's disease is reversal of the rectosigmoid ratio, ie. the rectum is narrower than the sigmoid colon. The rectum may have a 'saw tooth' appearance due to irregular muscle contractions.

Very short segment disease can be impossible to diagnose on a contrast enema as the transition point occurs too close to the anal canal to positively identify it. Total colonic Hirschsprung's may be impossible to differentiate from a microcolon and long segment disease from meconium plug syndrome. In all cases final positive diagnosis is made by means of suction mucosal biopsies (Fig. 13.5).

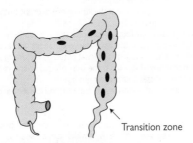

Transition zone

**Fig. 13.5** Hirchsprung's disease. Reversal of rectosigmoid ratio.

## Further reading

**1.** Berrocal T *et al.* (1999) Congenital anomalies of the small intestine, colon and rectum. *Radiographics* **19**; 1219–36.

# ⓘ **Necrotizing enterocolitis (NEC)**

## Aetiology

The cause of NEC is uncertain but mucosal damage, bacterial invasion and inflammatory responses all may lead to necrosis through bowel wall damage.

## Clinical features

- Occurs in premature neonates usually within the first 2 weeks of life.
- Abdominal distension.
- Bilious or blood stained nasogastric aspirates.
- Blood PR.
- Shock.
- Apnoea.
- Thrombocytopaenia.
- Neutropaenia.
- Acidosis.

## Imaging

### Radiographs: AXR

*Findings*

The appearances change as the disease develops as the features are transitory and not all stages are seen in every case. *The radiologist's role is to document progress and identify perforation.*

- Dilation of the bowel and mural thickening are present but alone are not sufficient to diagnose NEC.
- Rounded submucosal gas locules form causing a 'soap bubble' appearance. This may have the appearance of faeces within bowel but babies do not have adult-type faecal patterns for the first few weeks. Can occur anywhere from the oesophagus to the rectum but is commonest in the distal ileum and right colon.
- Extension of gas into the subserosal and intramuscular spaces causes linear bowel wall lucencies.
- Ascites.
- Gas bubbles pass through the portal venous system and become lodged in the portal veins in the liver, which can be seen as radiolucent branching structures. If present it is a sign of severe disease but it is not as grave as in the adult population.
- Perforation: Rigler's sign; outlining of the falciform ligament; lucency over the lateral aspect of the liver; subdiaphragmatic gas may be present. The 'continuous diaphragm sign' is caused but a large amount of free intraperitoneal gas outlining the peritoneal surface of the diaphragm from one lateral margin to the other. The 'football sign' is produced from a large pneumoperitoneum outlining the entire abdominal cavity. The bowel dilatation and intramural gas can make small locules of free intraperitoneal gas hard to appreciate. A horizontal beam lateral AXR (shoot-through lateral) with the patient remaining supine demonstrates triangular gas shapes lying under the anterior abdominal wall. These neonates are often very unstable and lateral decubitus positioning is not tolerated for long enough to allow gas to rise above the liver.

## Management

This is instigated on clinical suspicion even if the AXR is non-diagnostic and is usually conservative with IV antibiotics and TPN whilst stopping enteral feeding. Surgical treatment is reserved for cases involving perforation.

## Complications

Multiple strictures are the commonest complication. These can occur at any site previously affected and their number and extent are not related to the severity of the initial disease. Enterocysts (dilated segments of normal bowel between strictures), internal fistulas and adhesions can occur. Extensive surgical resections can result in too little bowel to adequately absorb nutrients leading to short bowel syndrome and malnutrition, dehydration and intractable diarrhoea.

## Further reading

1. Epelman M (2007) Necrotizing enterocolitis: review of state-of-the-art imaging findings with pathologic correlation. *RadioGraphics* **27**; 285–305.

# ⊙ Foreign body ingestion and inhalation

## Clinical features

- Commonest between 6 months and 3 years.
- Shortness of breath.
- Wheeze and stridor.
- Cough.
- Recurrent chest infections.
- Drooling.
- Refusing food.
- Vomiting.

## Location

Swallowed foreign bodies typically lodge within the oesophagus at sites of physiological stenosis: above cricopharyngeus, the aortic knuckle or at the gastro-oesophageal junction. Inhaled foreign bodies may lodge in the pharynx typically around the tonsils. Within the lungs they lodge in the lower lobe bronchi or right middle lobe bronchus.

## Types of foreign body

Coins are the commonest object. They, and other flat objects, lie with their long axis in the coronal plane in the oesophagus and the sagittal plane in the trachea. If a coin is present in the oesophagus for more than 24hrs it is unlikely to pass spontaneously and should be removed to prevent pressure necrosis.

Rounded objects that have reached the stomach are usually passed in 4–7 days without incident and if they lodge elsewhere consider pathological strictures, webs or rings.

Linear objects may impact at sites of sharp angulation such as the duodenum and ileocaecal valve.

Sharp objects should be removed to prevent peforation. Swallowed batteries should be removed endoscopically before they leave the stomach due to their poisonous content. Button batteries can be distinguished from coins by their stepped edge causing a double density rim. A single magnet is of little consequence but if more than one is swallowed bowel wall can get entrapped leading to pressure necrosis, perforation and fistula formation.

## Imaging strategies

An extended chest radiograph which includes the upper abdomen allows detection of swallowed and inhaled foreign bodies (if the history is unclear). The area of coverage can be reduced if there is a reliable history. A lateral neck view is helpful to exclude pharyngeal foreign bodies.

An inhaled foreign body in a bronchus acts as a ball valve. This may be the only sign of a radiolucent foreign body: lobar hyperexpansion causes increased lucency, reduction of lung markings and sometimes contralateral mediastinal shift.

If the CXR is normal and there is continuing clinical concern in an older cooperative child, an expiratory CXR may show air trapping within a lobe as persisting lucency and a failure to lose volume.

In younger infants, air trapping can be demonstrated by taking two lateral decubitus chest X-rays. The presence of air trapping will prevent that lung or lobe from compressing when it is in the dependent position.

# ① ② **Non-accidental injury**

When reporting paediatric radiographs, the possibility of non-accidental injury (NAI) should always be considered. The radiologist should ask the following questions:

- Does the injury on the radiograph seem appropriate for the history provided?
- Is a child of that age capable of doing what we are told they did?

*If you have any concerns then discuss the radiograph with a Consultant Radiologist with experience in this area and discuss the case with the clinicians.* This may provide more clinical information which may allay any suspicions, or alternatively it may alert the clinicians to a situation of which they were not aware. **Any final radiological report raising the possibility of NAI should not be written by a trainee alone.**

The role of radiology is to document the injuries present and to offer an opinion on the likely timing of injury and whether it is consistent with the mechanism of injury that has been suggested by the history.

If there is any concern by the emergency department regarding NAI the patient should be referred to the paediatricians. It is the responsibility of the paediatricians to review the history and examine the patient and if there is concern, admit the patient to the ward as a place of safety while further investigations are taking place.

## The skeletal survey

Once NAI is suspected it is common for a skeletal survey to be requested to document occult injuries and this is usually requested in younger children often below the age of 3. After this age, occult injury without other physical evidence or information from the child is not common enough to warrant whole body radiation exposure. A skeletal survey consists of a series of films covering both the axial and appendicular skeleton. A skeletal survey should be performed by two radiographers trained and experienced in paediatric radiography. It should always be performed during normal working hours and the films reviewed by a Consultant Radiologist with adequate training and experience before the patient leaves the department so any additional views can be performed. The films should be carefully reviewed by a Consultant Radiologist and in many institutions double reporting is practiced. The report should document all definite and suspected areas of injury and if the pattern of injury is highly suspicious of NAI this should also be commented upon. Delayed films may be of value in either dating injuries or demonstrating the development of callus at suspected sites of injury.

The plain film survey is complemented by a CT scan of the brain to document intracranial injuries. Skull fractures are surprisingly hard to identify on CT, even using thin slice reconstructions and bone reconstruction algorithms, and hence the skull radiographs should still be performed.

## Findings strongly associated with non accidental injuries

### Body fractures
- Posterior rib fractures.
- Multiple rib fractures.
- Scapular fractures.
- Acromial fractures.
- Pelvic fractures.
- Metaphyseal corner fractures.
- Multiple fractures of different ages.

### Skull fractures
- Bilateral.
- Crossing sutures.
- Branching or depressed fractures.

### Subdural haemorrhage location
- Parafalcine.
- Posterior fossa.
- Bilateral convexity.

## Further reading

**1.** British Society of Paediatric Radiology: Standard for skeletal surveys in suspected non-accidental injury (NAI) in children. http://www.bspr.org.uk/nai.htm.

**2.** Lonergan GJ, Baker AM, Morey MK *et al.* (2003) From the Archives of the AFIP Child Abuse: radiologic–pathologic correlation. *RadioGraphics* **23**; 811–45.

**3.** The Royal College of Radiologists and the Royal College of Paediatrics and Child Health (2008) *Intercollegiate Report from The Royal College of Radiologists and Royal College of Paediatrics and Child Health: Standards for Radiological Investigations of Suspected Non-accidental Injury* Royal College of Paediatrics and Child Health, London.

# Paediatric tube positions and complications

See also 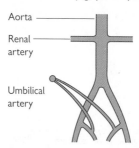 p. 106 for adult lines and tubes.

### Endotracheal tube

The tip should lie between C7 and T4 and above the carina. The small size of babies and neonates and the changes in position of the tube on head movement makes tube misplacement more common than in the adult population.

Intubation of a main bronchus leads to over ventilation of that lobe and increased risk of barotrauma and collapse of the non-ventilated lobe. If there is persistent collapse of the right upper lobe and the endotracheal tube appears correctly sited, then consider a tracheal bronchus.

The main long-term intubation risk is tracheal stenosis which is usually present in the subglottic region.

### Nasogastric tube

The tip of the nasogastric tube (NGT) should lie within the stomach and below the hemidiaphragm.

As the NGT has side holes, if the tip is just within the stomach these will lie in the distal oesophagus risking aspiration of medication or feed.

If the tube is inserted too distally, the tip can pass into the duodenum which may lead to bilious aspiration and an erroneous diagnosis of obstruction.

Long-term tubes can erode through the gastric wall.

### Umbilical arterial catheter (UAC)

This can be distinguished from other lines due to its initial inferior course from the umbilicus as the catheter passes through the umbilical artery. In the pelvis it deviates superiorly as it enters one of the common iliac arteries and then reaches the aorta (Fig. 13.6).

The tip should lie either at T6–T10 (high position) or at L3–L5 (low).

Aorta

Renal artery

Umbilical artery

**Fig. 13.6** The umbilical arteries.

*Complications*

Thrombosis can occlude the iliac vessels or aorta and emboli can form. Positioning the line at T10 or L3 increases the risk of occluding thrombus or emboli entering the main spinal or splanchnic arteries.

The line can cause irritation to the vascular endothelium and this can eventually lead to stricturing.

## Umbilical venous catheter (UVC)

In contrast to the UAC, this catheter deviates superiorly on immediately passing though the umbilicus. It passes through the umbilical vein to reach the left portal vein. From there it enters the ductus venosus which it passes through towards the inferior vena cava.

The tip should lie at T9–T10.

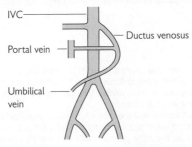

**Fig. 13.7** The umbilical vein.

### Complications

- Deviation into the hepatic veins or portal veins can cause hepatic haematoma, ischaemia and necrosis. Occlusion of the portal vein can lead to portal hypertension.
- If the tip is intracardiac, arrhythmias may result and it can even penetrate through the myocardium to reach the pericardial space.
- If the line is inserted too distally it can pass through the tricuspid valve to enter the pulmonary arteries. Alternatively it can pass through a patent foramen ovale into the left atrium and then into the pulmonary veins.
- Inferior vena cava (IVC) thrombosis can occur with emboli formation.
- Endothelial irritation can cause stricture formation.

### Scalp lines

Long line access sites are commonly in the antecubital fossae or the inguinal regions. Insertion of these lines may be difficult because of their small calibre and damage from previous attempts. Scalp lines are inserted if peripheral access fails. The superficial temporal and posterior auricular veins are commonly used. These often have a tortuous course and the tip should lie within the jugular veins or more centrally.

### Further reading

**1.** Narla LD, Hom M, Lofland GK *et al.* (1991) Evaluation of umbilical catheter and tube placement in premature infants. *RadioGraphics* **11**; 849–63.

# ⑦ **Hypertrophic pyloric stenosis**

Hypertrophy of the pyloric sphincter causing gastric outlet obstruction.

## Clinical features

- Typically presents at 2–8 weeks.
- Projectile vomiting immediately after food.
- Weight loss.
- Failure to thrive.
- Palpable mass (often described as an 'olive') in the subhepatic region.
- Alkalosis.

## Imaging

### US

*Protocol*

- Standard abdominal US using an 8–10MHz curvilinear probe.
- Focused US of the upper abdomen using 10–12MHz linear probe.
- The pylorus is usually in the midline inferior to the liver but can be displaced by a very full stomach.
- The pylorus is best seen if the stomach contains clear fluid and this also allows assessment of pyloric opening. The patient typically has a nasogastric tube and if the pylorus is difficult to find try giving water (not milk as this has a slower gastric transit time) if the stomach is empty or aspirating if full.

*Findings*

The pylorus is thickened and enlongated. The muscle wall is hypoechoic and the mucosa is hyperechoic. Exaggerated peristaltic waves are seen in the stomach but the pylorus does not open. Scan longitudinally and transversly to measure the length and muscle wall thickness (from serosa to mucosa); Fig. 13.8.

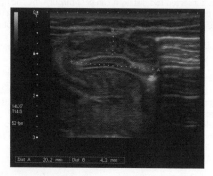

**Fig. 13.8** Transverse ultrasound image demonstrating pyloric stenosis: distance A represents the canal length; B is the muscle thickness.

*Measurements*
- Normal pylorus length <15mm.
- Normal muscle wall thickness <3mm.

Wall thickening is the most sensitive measurement.

## Further reading

**1.** Rohrschneider W et al. (1998) Pyloric muscle in asymptomatic infants: sonographic evaluation and discrimination from idiopathic hypertrophic pyloric stenosis. *Pediatr Radiol* **28**; 429–34.

## ⚙ ⓘ **Paediatric trauma**

# Imaging of blunt abdominal trauma

The choice of imaging modality should depend on the nature of the trauma, when it occurred, and the stability of the patient.

An unstable patient with recent trauma usually requires urgent CT. If there is a delayed presentation, the patient is well and the trauma is minor then ultrasound assessment should be the first line.

As in adult cases, emergency life-saving surgery should not be delayed by imaging.

See also 📖 p. 184 for adult abdominal trauma.

### US

Abdominal ultrasound in children is a highly effective modality. Their size and lack of intra-abdominal fat allows the use of high-frequency probes, giving excellent spatial resolution.

*Protocol*

- Use both 6–10MHz curvilinear and 8–12MHz linear probes.
- Perform a thorough assessment of each solid organ including Doppler interrogation.
- Review the retroperitoneum for haematomas.
- Look for free fluid in the abdomen and pelvis.

*Findings*

Haematomas are seen as hypoechoic areas when acute, becoming more echoic as they organize. They have a linear configuration in a laceration, rounded as a focal haematoma or biconvex when subcapsular. Doppler assessment of each organ may reveal areas of absent flow suggesting injury. Retroperitoneal haematomas are best seen by looking for displacement of normal structures such as the kidneys, aorta and IVC. Free fluid should be easily identified which is always abnormal; the exception is a small amount of fluid in the pouch of Douglas in post-pubertal girls.

A normal well-performed ultrasound with good views of the organs effectively excludes a serious intra-abdominal injury requiring urgent surgical intervention. Small liver and splenic lacerations may not be identified, however the current surgical trend is towards conservative management of these in stable patients. It must be remembered that the clinicians must treat the patient and not the scan results. If there is a change in the patient's condition then the patient must be reassessed clinically and, if appropriate, reimaged using either ultrasound or CT.

### CT

*Protocol*

Low-dose CT protocols should be selected which use low tube currents and modulate the exposure based on the density of the body part being examined. Exact scanning parameters depend on the manufacturer of the CT and the age of the patient. Modern machines have a selection of paediatric protocols: choose one that is appropriate for both the patient's age and size.

- Scan from diaphragm to the symphysis. Only include the chest if there are specific concerns within the thorax which cannot be addressed with a CXR.
- IV contrast 2ml/kg. This can be given by hand injection or via a pump at 1–2ml/s with acquisition at 60s. Pre contrast and arterial phase images are not routinely obtained. If there is specific concern regarding a vascular injury, discuss the scan with a senior paediatric radiologist.
- A small amount of oral contrast medium may be given.
- 2.5mm reconstructions with a soft tissue algorithm and 1–1.25mm with a bone algorithm.

*Findings*

- Look for free fluid or gas within the peritoneum.
- Assess each solid organ for low attenuation areas such as linear laceration, rounded haematomas or areas of avascularity. Pay attention to the pancreas as this can be crushed in handlebar injuries.
- The presence of contrast in the duodenum may help in detecting a filling defect caused by an intramural haematoma which is also common in handlebar injuries.
- Use thin slice reconstructions and MPRs to look for fractures and to assess the spine.
- Look at the lung bases for pneumothoraces.

# Cervical spinal trauma

Children under 8 years of age have fewer injuries then those over 8 year years old. They are predominantly found in the upper cervical spine and ligamentous injuries are more common than fractures. This is due to the head being proportionally heavier, ligamentous laxity and the horizontal orientation of the facet joints in children. In older children the injuries are predominantly fractures in the lower cervical spine. In most cases, good plain films are capable of clearing the cervical spine.

See also 📖 p. 254 for adult spinal trauma imaging.

## Imaging

### Radiographs of the cervical spine

*Protocol*

Include the skull base and T1 on the lateral view. Use a swimmer's view or oblique film if cervicothoracic junction is not visible.

*Findings*

- Normal prevertebral soft tissues in children:
  - C1–C4 <7mm (<½ AP vertebral body diameter).
  - C4–C7 <14mm (<1 AP vertebral body diameter).
  - Unreliable if intubated and can be increased by crying. Remember the relatively increased size of the tonsils and adenoids in children.
  - Normal soft tissues cannot exclude a fracture, especially of the posterior elements.

*Alignment*

The anterior and posterior spinal lines, and spinolaminar line should be smooth. The relatively large head of a child often leads to immobilization of the neck in a flexed position on a spinal board.

*Atlanto-occipital dislocation*

This can be assessed using the following ratio, which if greater than one, indicates dislocation:

$$\text{Powers ratio} = \frac{\text{Basion to posterior arch distance}}{\text{Opisthion to anterior arch distance}}$$

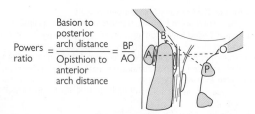

$$\text{Powers ratio} = \frac{\text{Basion to posterior arch distance}}{\text{Opisthion to anterior arch distance}} = \frac{BP}{AO}$$

**Fig. 13.9** The Powers ratio: if greater than 1 this indicates atlanto–axial dislocation. This is demonstrated on a schematic showing the landmarks on a lateral C-spine radiograph. A: anterior arch of the atlas; O: opisthion; B: basion; P: posterior arch (spinolaminar line) of atlas; ratio = BP/AO.

*Atlanto–axial subluxation*

- Atlanto–axial distance >5mm
- <2mm change from extended to flexed

*C2/3 pseudosubluxation*

Physiological anterior subluxation of C2 on C3 is common up to the age of 8 and can occur in the early teens. A flexed immobilization position accentuates the appearance of the pseudosubluxation. Look at a straight line connecting the anterior border of the posterior arch of C1 and C3. This should pass within 2mm of the anterior cortex of the posterior arch of C2. An increased distance indicates a true injury may be present (Fig. 13.10).

*C1 Pseudospread*

There is pseudospread of C1 with the lateral masses overhanging C2 on the peg view. This is common under 4 years and decreases with age. The odontoid peg is centrally placed and there is symmetrical overhang of up to 3mm.

Traumatic Subluxation    Pseudosubluxation

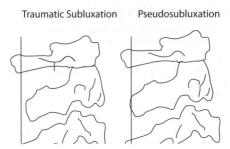

**Fig. 13.10** Traumatic vs pseudosubluxation of C2/3.

*Fractures*

Remember that each vertebra forms from several ossification centres and the cartilaginous bone and synchondroses should not be confused with fractures. A fracture line is not corticated unlike synchondroses.

Commonest areas of concern are the os terminale at the tip of the odontoid peg (ossifies at 3–6yrs and fuses at 12yrs), the synchondrosis between C2 body and odontoid peg (fuses between 3–6yrs but visible until 11yrs), and the ring apophyses (ossify at 10–12yrs and fuse at 25yrs). If there is any doubt, then refer to an atlas of normal variants or an experienced paediatric radiologist.

*CT*

If the abnormal plain film radiographs are of good quality and the child has been examined by an experienced trauma surgeon it may be possible to limit a CT to a specific area to reduce the radiation dose to the thyroid. In the intubated and ventilated patient it may not be possible and the entire cervical spine should be imaged.

*Protocol*

- Select a low-dose paediatric spine protocol.
- Unenhanced study
- 0.5–1mm reconstructions using both bone and soft tissue algorithms.

*Findings*

*Review Areas:* Use MPRs to review the data in axial, coronal and sagittal planes to assess the alignment. Remember that each vertebra forms from several ossification centres and the cartilaginous bone and synchondroses should not be confused with fractures. A fracture line is not corticated unlike synchondroses.

## Further reading

**1.** Akgür FM, Aktug T, Olguner M *et al.* (1997) Prospective study investigating routine usage of ultrasonography as the initial diagnostic modality for the evaluation of children sustaining blunt abdominal trauma. *Journal of Trauma–Injury Infection and Critical Care* **42(4)**; 626–8.

**2.** Lustrin ES, Karakas SP, Ortiz AO *et al.* (2003) Pediatric cervical spine: normal anatomy, variants, and trauma. *RadioGraphics* **23**; 539–60.

# ⑦ Posterior urethral valves

Smooth muscle and connective tissue structures within the membranous and prostatic parts of the male urethra.

## Classification

- *Young Type I*. Commonest: arise from verumontanum extending distally to lateral walls of the urethra due to abnormal integration of Wolffian ducts into the urethra.
- *Young Type II*. Rarest: longitudinal folds from verumontanum to the bladder neck
- *Young Type III*. Rare: diaphragm with central hole at the level of the verumontanum due to failure of canalization of the cloacal membrane.

## Clinical features

Increased intravesical pressure is required to overcome the valve. This leads to bladder wall hypertrophy, increased bladder volume and retrograde flow of urine through the vesicoureteric junctions into the ureters. Increased pressure in the ureters causes hydronephrosis and reflux increases risk of pyelonephritis secondary to a lower urinary tract infection and scarring of the kidneys. Clinical presentation includes the following:

- Antenatal diagnosis of large keyhole-shaped bladder, usually with hydronephrosis.
- Urinary tract infections.
- Poor stream.
- Abnormal renal function.

## Imaging

### Ultrasound

*Protocol*

Routine abdominal ultrasound using 6–10MHz curvilinear probe depending on patent size. Prone imaging of kidneys with both curvilinear and 8–10MHz linear probe to assess renal size, corticomedullary differentiation and urothelial thickening.

*Findings*

- Hydronephrosis and hydroureters which are usually bilateral but often asymmetrical in appearance.
- Large volume bladder with thickened and trabeculated wall.
- Dilated posterior urethra.

Estimated bladder volume in ml = (Age in years + 2) × 30

Normal bladder wall thickness ≤3mm when full.

### Micturating cystourethrogram (MCUG)

Usually performed in patients under 1 year old. After this age the patient will remember this as a traumatic experience. If suspected in older children, discuss the possibility of cystoscopy and suprapubic catheterization under general anaesthetic (GA) with the paediatric urology team.

*Protocol*

Place the patient supine on the screening table on several absorbent pads. Insert a 6 Fr urinary catheter and secure in position with tape.

Starting in the supine position, instill warmed water-soluble contrast, such as urografin 150, into the bladder via an IV giving set from an elevated bottle of contrast medium. A syringe can be used but the drip method prevents over distension of the urinary tract. Using low-dose intermittent pulsed fluoroscopy, a fluoroscopic image of early bladder filling should be saved to demonstrate filling defects from ureterocoeles. Turn patient into a 45° lateral position to allow visualization of the posterior urethra.

Continue filling the bladder and store a second image grab of a full bladder to demonstrate bladder shape and trabeculation if present. Continue filling until voiding occurs. Take an exposure of the entire urethra from bladder to penile tip with the catheter *in situ*. Observe the posterior bladder wall for contrast medium within the ureters: if it is present in the ureters at any stage image the kidneys to document the level of the reflux.

Remove the contrast medium-covered pads and fill the bladder for a second voiding cycle. This second cycle permits better bladder filling and demonstrates more reflux than a single cycle. The catheter may act as a urethral stent holding open the valve and therefore during filling, loosen the securing tape and when voiding begins quickly remove the catheter and take a urethral exposure. This may reveal valves not seen on the first voiding cycle.

Once voiding has finished remove the contrast medium-covered pads, turn the baby supine and take a cross-kidney exposure to document reflux.

*Findings*

Dilated posterior urethra compared to the penile urethra with sharp tapering. The valve is seen as a thin linear filling defect usually arising from the anterior wall of the urethra. Reflux may be present and is often bilateral and asymmetrical.

**Further reading**

**1.** Agrawalla S, Pearce R, Goodman TR (2004) How to perform the perfect voiding cystourethrogram. *Pediatr Radiol* **34**; 114–19.

**2.** Levin T *et al.* (2007) Congenital anomalies of the male urethra. *Pediatr Radiol* **37**; 851–62.

# ① ? **Irritable hip**

The commonest cause is reactive synovitis but septic arthritis, which can cause rapid joint damage, needs to be excluded.

## Clinical features

- Painful hip.
- Limping or refusing to weight-bear on one leg.
- Low grade fever.
- Leucocytosis.

## Imaging strategy

### Radiographs of the hip

AP pelvis to exclude a fracture, arthropathy or bone destruction. If there is clinical concern about a slipped upper femoral epiphysis (SUFE) then a frog lateral view is advised. If the hip radiograph is normal and there is a history of trauma in a patient who is unable to indicate the site of pain then radiographs of the rest of the leg should be performed to look for fractures.

### US

#### Protocol

Hips effusions are best seen in the synovial reflection anterior to the neck of the femur. Image using a 6–12MHz linear probe in the sagittal plane parallel to the neck of the femur. Always compare with the other side and record the maximum depth of fluid. Document the Doppler flow in the synovium. Try to image the affected hip in the neutral, internally and externally rotated positions.

#### Findings

- Anechoic or echogenic biconvex fluid collection between the femoral neck and the joint capsule.
- Normal joint capsule thickness is 3–7mm and there may be up to 2mm difference between the hips.
- Doppler assessment may show increased Doppler flow in the synovium but this does not reliably differentiate septic and reactive arthritis.
- Synovial hypertrophy can look like an effusion with low level echoes from debris. Rotating the hip internally and externally can cause the synovium to move and bring true fluid into view.

## Management

There are no ultrasound criteria to definitely confirm that a joint effusion is not infected and if the clinical findings are compatible (e.g. fever and raised inflammatory markers) then septic arthritis should be assumed. Local policies regarding the further management vary and these should be followed.

Many authorities recommend immediate formal joint washout in theatre in all cases of suspected septic arthritis in the presence of a joint effusion. The fluid is sent for microbiological culture and the joint washed clean.

Some suggest joint aspiration and fluid microscopy prior to washout. Aspiration can be performed under ultrasound guidance using sedation or under general anaesthetic in theatre. This may reduce the need for formal washout of the joint, but many orthopaedic surgeons prefer to proceed directly to definitive treatment given the potential risk of the microscopy producing a false-negative result.

Aspiration in the radiology department under ultrasound guidance is also controversial: it is performed in some centres but the general consensus is against this practice. Often there is insufficient staff trained to safely sedate the child and without sedation the procedure can become painful and traumatic for the patient even when local anesthetic is used; under these conditions a sterile field cannot be maintained. However, some have argued that aspirating the joint, even in the absence of septic arthritis, may relieve the symptoms which are primarily caused by stretching of the joint capsule.

**Further reading**

**1.** Fang C, Portess H and Wilson D (2004) Application of ultrasound in the diagnosis and management of paediatric hip conditions. *Current Orthopaedics* **18**; 291–303.

# Interventional radiology

Dinkuke Warakaulle

# Introduction

Information obtained from cross-sectional imaging is crucial for planning many interventional radiological procedures. Cross-sectional imaging has largely replaced invasive diagnostic procedures.

## Checklist for all interventional radiology procedures

- Full blood count (platelet count should be >100x10$^9$/L).
- Coagulation profile (INR<1.5 for most procedures or <2.5 for venous procedures such as caval filter placement).
- Heparin infusions are usually stopped 1hr before the procedure. Low molecular weight heparin injections should be stopped 24hrs before. These steps may not be possible if the patient has a prosthetic heart valve.
- Serum creatinine, urea and electrolytes. If there is evidence of renal impairment and intravascular iodinated contrast is to be used during the procedure, the patient should be pre-hydrated with intravenous fluids if possible.
- Review diagnostic imaging and plan procedure.
- Obtain informed consent. The person performing the procedure should obtain informed consent whenever possible. However, this may be delegated to another clinician who is suitably qualified and has appropriate training.[1]
- Ensure that the patient has suitable intravenous access.
- Ensure that the patient is stable. Anaesthetic support may be needed.
- Adequate analgesia should be provided. Most interventional procedures can be performed with good local anaesthesia (usually 1% lidocaine without adrenaline, infiltrated into the skin and subcutaneous tissues to a maximum volume of 10mls), but some procedures, such as nephrostomy placement, require intravenous sedation and analgesia (📖 p. 32).
- A small skin inscision is then made with a scalpel, which should be of sufficient size to admit the largest sheath or catheter that is to be inserted.

# Chest drain

## Indication

- Urgent chest drain placement under image guidance is usually for the drainage of an empyema.
- Empyema has to be differentiated from a simple parapneumonic effusion, as the latter does not require drainage.

## Imaging

### US

*Findings*

US features of empyema:
- Echogenic effusion
- Loculated effusion (internal septation on US)
- Gas-containing effusion (internal echoes, 'comet-tail' artefact)

### CT

*Findings*

CT features of empyema:
- Loculated effusion (multiple gas locules)
- Enhancing pleural layers
- Inflammatory streaking of the extrapleural fat

See Fig. 14.1.

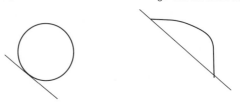

Lung abscess
Acute angle with the chest wall

Empyema
Obtuse angle with the chest wall

**Fig. 14.1** Differentiation of lung abscess and empyema.

If there is a simple effusion on US and CT, the decision to place a chest drain is made on the basis of a pleural pH of <7.2 on a diagnostic aspirate.[2]

A peripheral lung abscess must be differentiated from an empyema, as a chest drain placed into the former can result in a bronchopleural fistula.

| Lung abscess | Empyema |
| --- | --- |
| Acute angle with chest wall | Obtuse angle with chest wall |
| Destroys adjacent lung so usually no collapse | Compresses and collapses adjacent lung |
| | Split pleura sign—the effusion separates the 2 pleural layers |

## Technique

- See checklist 📖 p. 372.
- Sterile technique is used.
- US guidance is preferred. A linear transducer with a wide-angle beam and small footprint (as used for echocardiography) is ideal for most US-guided procedures, especially thoracic interventions, as it allows easy access between ribs. Curvilinear abdominal transducers can also be used.
- Ideally, the patient should be positioned sitting up, and leaning slightly forwards, to maximize separation of the posterior and lateral ribs.
- The collection is located using US. A suitable approach is selected. This should be at least a hand breadth lateral to the midline, and should skirt the upper border of an overlying rib. Adhering to these principles minimizes the risk of damaging the intercostal vessels.
- A 16 G sheathed needle (e.g. Abbocath, Abbott, Sligo, Republic of Ireland) with a 10ml syringe attached is advanced into the collection. This is best done under US guidance for small collections, but can be done 'blindly' after marking the access point on the skin for larger collections.
- Suction is applied to the syringe as the needle is advanced. When fluid is aspirated, the needle is held still at that point, and the sheath is advanced further into the collection, until a stable position is obtained. The initial aspirate is sent for microbiological analysis. The needle is removed, and the sheath left in place. Placing a finger over the sheath hub at this time minimizes the risk of air entry into the pleural space.
- A short, stiff guidewire (e.g. Amplatz Extra Stiff 80cm, Cook, Bloomington, USA) is then advanced into the collection. When a good length of wire has passed through the sheath, serial dilatation of the tract is performed to allow passage of a pigtail (locking or non-locking) catheter into the collection. A drain size of 10–12 Fr is required.
- The drain is secured to the skin with adhesive dressings, and connected to a drainage bag. An underwater seal may be used for chest drains, but is not mandatory in this particular setting.
- When documenting the procedure in the clinical notes, it should be specified if a locking pigtail drain has been used, as this needs to be unlocked before removal.

# Nephrostomy

**Nephrostomy for acute or acute-on-chronic renal failure**

*Indication*

Hydronephrosis will have been established on diagnostic imaging prior to the request for nephrostomy. If there is bilateral hydronephrosis, it is usually sufficient to drain one kidney in the emergency setting, provided there is no evidence of sepsis. The kidney which is more normal-sized, with greater cortical thickness on diagnostic imaging, is drained preferentially.

**Nephrostomy for sepsis associated with an obstructed kidney**

- Requires urgent nephrostomy placement.

**Technique**

- See checklist 📖 p. 372.
- In addition to the pre-procedure checks mentioned previously, the serum potassium level should be specifically checked. Significant hyperkalaemia should be treated prior to the procedure, as it carries a risk of cardiac arrest. The requirement for treating hyperkalaemia depends on whether it is of acute or chronic onset. If the serum potassium is elevated, discussion with the referring clinician as to whether treatment of this is necessary before the procedure is recommended.
- Nephrostomy is usually performed under antibiotic cover (ciprofloxacin 500mg orally or co-amoxiclav 1.2g iv).
- The patient is positioned semi-prone, with the side undergoing intervention upwards.
- Sterile technique is used.
- Under US guidance, posterior mid or lower pole calyx is punctured—via a posterior approach to minimize vascular injury—using a 22 G needle from a percutaneous access set (e.g. Skater Introducer Set, PBN Medicals, Stenløse, Denmark). Direct puncture of the renal pelvis should be avoided as this has a higher risk of vascular injury.
- When the needle tip is seen in the collecting system, a connecting tube with a tap and syringe half-filled with contrast medium is connected to the needle hub, after first flushing the tube with contrast.
- Aspiration is performed through the syringe, to confirm that the needle is within the collecting system, which is then opacified with contrast. Care should be taken to avoid over-distension, to avoid rupture and/or dissemination of infective organisms.
- The 0.018in Mandril wire of the access set is then passed through the needle. Fluoroscopy is used to confirm that a good length of the stiff part of the wire is within the collecting system, and that it has a stable position (ideally, looped into an upper pole calyx).
- The three-part dilator is then passed over the wire under fluoroscopic guidance. The dilator should be pushed along the line of the wire, which should not be allowed to kink. The inner metal core of the dilator is only needed to penetrate the renal capsule, and should be

held back once this has been achieved. The outer dilator is pushed into the collecting system.

- The metal and plastic stiffeners are removed, and a short stiff guidewire is then advanced into the collecting system parallel to the Mandril wire.
- The dilator is then removed, leaving both wires *in situ*.
- Serial dilatation of the tract is performed over the stiff wire. The Mandril wire is left *in situ* as a 'safety' to maintain access in case the stiff wire falls out.
- The pigtail nephrostomy catheter is advanced over the stiff wire into a stable position within the collecting system (ideally with the pigtail formed in an upper pole calyx). The Mandril wire is now removed, and the nephrostomy catheter is secured to the skin with sutures or adhesive dressings.
- The catheter is connected to a drainage bag. Active aspiration should not be performed, as rapid decompression can lead to bleeding.
- A single-pass technique using a pigtail catheter mounted on a trocar (e.g. Skater Single Step Drainage Set, PBN Medicals, Stenløse, Denmark) under US guidance can be used, particularly if the collecting system is greatly dilated. This has the advantage of reducing the risk of bacteraemia by minimizing manipulation, but can be technically more challenging.

# Abdominal and pelvic drain insertion

### Indication
Usually for patients with abdominal or pelvic collections seen on diagnostic imaging with associated signs of sepsis and failure to respond to antibiotic therapy.

### Technique
- See checklist 📖 p. 372.
- The technique is similar to that described for chest drain insertion, although the procedure is almost always performed under direct image guidance.
- CT with intravenous, and if possible oral, contrast medium is the diagnostic investigation of choice. Drainage can be performed at the same time.
- Superficial collections can be drained under US guidance, provided that interposed bowel can be confidently excluded.
- Deep pelvic collections may be drained with the patient prone via a posterior approach. Whenever possible, an approach inferior to the piriformis muscle and as close as possible to the sacrum is preferable, as this minimizes the risk of injury to the sciatic nerve and gluteal vessels. See Fig. 14.2.
- 10–12 French locking pigtail drains are usually used for these procedures.

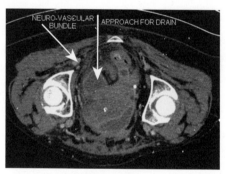

**Fig. 14.2** Prone approach for CT-guided pelvic drain.

# Percutaneous aspiration

Thoracic and abdominal collections can also be aspirated under imaging guidance for diagnostic or therapeutic purposes. Diagnostic aspiration can usually be performed with a standard 21 G needle, or with a 22 G spinal needle for deeper collections. Therapeutic aspiration to dryness of a small collection may require a larger sheathed needle such as an Abbocath.

# Cholecystostomy

## Indications

- Acute cholecystitis which fails to settle despite 48hrs of intravenous antibiotics
- Acute cholecystits in patients who are high-risk cases for emergency surgery
- Gallbladder empyema
- Sepsis in critically ill patients, where there is no other obvious source of infection, and there is a possibility of acalculous cholecysitis, even if no gallstones are seen on US

## Technique[3]

- See checklist ☐ p. 372.
- Sterile technique is used.
- The gallbladder is located using US, and a sheathed needle with attached syringe is passed into it under US guidance. A transhepatic route is generally favoured for needle placement, as this is thought to minimize the risk of bile leak. However, there is no strong evidence to favour this practice. See Fig. 14.3.

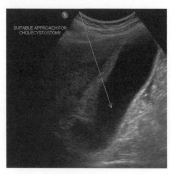

**Fig. 14.3** Approach for US-guided cholecystostomy.

- Suction is applied to the syringe as the needle is advanced. When bile (or pus) is aspirated, needle tip position within the gallbladder is confirmed on US. Large volumes should not be aspirated, as collapsing the gallbladder makes drain placement more difficult. The aspirated sample should be sent for microbiological analysis.
- The needle is then held still, and the sheath is advanced into a stable position.
- A short stiff guidewire is passed through the sheath. A good position within the gallbladder is confirmed when the wire is seen to loop within the gall bladder on fluoroscopy.
- Serial dilatation of the tract with pigtail drain placement is then performed as previously described.

# IVC filter placement

### Indications

There is currently no strong evidence base for the clinical indications or outcomes for caval filter placement. Probably the only generally accepted indication is recent proximal deep vein thrombosis (DVT) with an absolute contraindication to anticoagulation.

However, filters are placed for more controversial indications such as thromboembolism in patients at high risk of bleeding (but not currently bleeding), recurrent thromboembolism despite full anticoagulation, extensive DVT or DVT with a free-floating proximal end.

### Technique[4]

- If both femoral veins are occluded by thrombus, an internal jugular vein approach is used for placement.
- An initial cavogram is performed to exclude caval thrombus, determine the position of the renal veins (usually seen as filling defects in the IVC due to inflow of unpacified blood) and to measure the caval diameter at the site of placement, which should not exceed the manufacturer's recommendation.
- The optimum position for the filter is with its upper end at the level of, but no higher than, the inflow from the lowermost renal vein. The filter should lie with its long axis parallel to the long axis of the IVC.

# Acute limb ischaemia

### Aetiology and clinical features

The commonest cause of acute limb ischaemia is *in situ* thrombus formation or impaction of an embolus that originated elsewhere in the circulatory system. Both of these usually occur at the site of a pre-existing stenosis. Emboli also commonly lodge at arterial branch points such as the popliteal trifurcation.

Similar events can also occur in haemodialysis fistulas, where the diagnosis is clinically evident, although it can be confirmed with Doppler US if necessary.

Aortic dissection as a cause of limb ischaemia should be considered in patients:
- with a suggestive clinical history
- with no previous predisposing conditions such as peripheral vascular disease or atrial fibrillation
- with arm ischaemia, especially bilateral
- with arm and leg ischaemia
- with limb ischaemia and new focal neurology

### Imaging

Diagnostic imaging (Doppler US, CT or MR angiography) is mandatory in acute limb ischaemia to establish the level and extent of occlusion.

Diagnostic catheter angiography is only required in special situations (e.g. limb ischaemia following trauma, where digital subtraction angiography is the only imaging modality with sufficient spatial resolution to detect small dissection flaps), or for non-diagnostic cross-sectional studies.

Aortic dissection should be investigated with CT angiography (📖 p. 114).

### Management

*Treatment options for acute limb ischaemia*
- Surgical embolectomy.
- Percutaneous thrombectomy: requires specialized endovascular devices.
- Intra-arterial thrombolysis: requires a high-dependency unit (HDU) facility for monitoring and facilities to perform frequent repeat angiograms to assess progression of treatment.

*Contraindications to thrombolysis*
- Absolute: stroke or recent transient ischaemic attack (TIA), active or recent bleeding, significant coagulopathy.
- Relative: recent (<3 months) neurosurgery or head injury, recent (<10 days) resuscitation, surgery or trauma, uncontrolled hypertension (systolic >180mmHg, diastolic >110mmHg), recent arterial puncture, intracranial tumour, recent eye surgery.
- Minor: pregnancy, endocarditis, haemorrhagic diabetic retinopathy, liver failure with coagulopathy.

# Phlegmasia cerulea dolens: venous thrombosis

Specific condition which presents with a swollen, painful, cyanotic limb, which can proceed to venous gangrene. There is an association with malignancy, and the morbidity and mortality of this condition are significant.

The pathophysiology is of extensive venous thrombosis, which also involves the post-capillary venules. Surgical thrombectomy therefore has a low rate of limb salvage.

The treatment, favoured by many clinicians, is thrombolytic therapy delivered *intra-arterially*, so that the agent diffuses into the occluded venules.

# Bleeding

### Definition and aetiology

Intractable bleeding that requires imaging to locate the source and/or radiological intervention. It is usually due to one of the following:

- Spontaneous gastrointestinal bleeding
- Trauma
- Post-surgery
- Post-partum

Haemorrhage from visceral arteries can occur into following compartments:

- Intraluminal
- Intraperitoneal
- Retroperitoneal

### Imaging

#### CT

MDCT angiography is the investigation of choice. It has a similar sensitivity to catheter angiography for the detection of gastro-intestinal bleeding, and can detect bleeding rates of 0.5ml/min.[5] A 3-phase protocol with image acquisition in the pre-contrast, arterial and delayed (70s post injection) phases is required.

When evaluating CT images, it is important to distinguish free fluid from intra-abdominal haematoma, as the latter should prompt a search for a source. CT features of haematoma:

- Similar attenuation (approximately 40–60HU) to skeletal muscle on CECT.
- High attenuation (approx 40HU) on NECT.
- Layering with time ('haematocrit effect').
- Visible active extravasation of contrast on arterial phase images.

### Management

#### Treatment of haemorrhage

In addition to the pre-procedure checklist mentioned previously, special attention should be given to correcting any coagulopathy in bleeding patients prior to embolization, which will maximize the efficacy of the procedure.

The choice of embolic material depends on the clinical scenario:

- Metal coils are used to occlude arteries causing intraluminal gastrointestinal bleeding and for other intra-abdominal visceral arterial haemorrhages.
- Gelatin sponge can be delivered as pledgets or as a slurry. It causes reversible arterial occlusion, and is favoured in situations such as postpartum haemorrhage and to embolize bleeding branches of the internal iliac arteries in pelvic trauma.
- Microspheres can be used to embolize bleeding tumours such as hepatomas.

Rupture of larger arteries can be treated with covered stent-grafts.

Even if embolization is not technically feasible, it may be possible to achieve temporary haemostasis by balloon occlusion of the supplying artery, to stabilize the patient before definitive treatment.

## Further reading

**1.** Standards for patient consent particular to radiology. *RCR* 2005.

**2.** Heffner JE, Brown LK, Barbieri C and Deleo JM (1995) Plewal fluid chemical analysis in parapneumonic effusions: a meta-analysis. *Am J Respir Crit Care Med* **151**; 1700–8.

**3.** Boland GW, Lee MJ, Leving J and Mueller PR (1994) Percutaneous cholecytogramy in cirtically ill patients: easy response and final outcome in 82 patients. *AJR* **163**; 339–42.

**4.** The thrombosis interest group of Canada. Clinical guide: IVC filters. http://www.tigc.org/pdf/venacava04.pdf

**5.** Kuhle WE and Sheiman RG (2003) Detection of Active Colonic Haemorrhage with use of Helical CT: findings in a swine model. *Radiology* **228**(3); 743–52.

# Index